SpringerBriefs in Electrical and Computer Engineering

Speech Technology

Series Editor
Amy Neustein

Editor's Note

The authors of this series have been hand selected. They comprise some of the most outstanding scientists—drawn from academia and private industry—whose research is marked by its novelty, applicability, and practicality in providing broad-based speech solutions. The Springer Briefs in Speech Technology series provides the latest findings in speech technology gleaned from comprehensive literature reviews and *empirical investigations* that are performed in both laboratory and *real life* settings. Some of the topics covered in this series include the presentation of real life commercial deployment of spoken dialog systems, contemporary methods of speech parameterization, developments in information security for automated speech, forensic speaker recognition, use of sophisticated speech analytics in call centers, and an exploration of new methods of soft computing for improving human–computer interaction. Those in academia, the private sector, the self service industry, law enforcement, and government intelligence are among the principal audience for this series, which is designed to serve as an important and essential reference guide for speech developers, system designers, speech engineers, linguists, and others. In particular, a major audience of readers will consist of researchers and technical experts in the automated call center industry where speech processing is a key component to the functioning of customer care contact centers.

Amy Neustein, Ph.D., serves as editor in chief of the *International Journal of Speech Technology* (Springer). She edited the recently published book *Advances in Speech Recognition: Mobile Environments, Call Centers and Clinics* (Springer 2010), and serves as quest columnist on speech processing for Womensenews. Dr. Neustein is the founder and CEO of Linguistic Technology Systems, a NJbased think tank for intelligent design of advanced natural language-based emotion detection software to improve human response in monitoring recorded conversations of terror suspects and helpline calls.

Dr. Neustein's work appears in the peer review literature and in industry and mass media publications. Her academic books, which cover a range of political, social, and legal topics, have been cited in the Chronicles of Higher Education and have won her a pro Humanitate Literary Award. She serves on the visiting faculty of the National Judicial College and as a plenary speaker at conferences in artificial intelligence and computing. Dr. Neustein is a member of MIR (machine intelligence research) Labs, which does advanced work in computer technology to assist underdeveloped countries in improving their ability to cope with famine, disease/illness, and political and social affliction. She is a founding member of the New York City Speech Processing Consortium, a newly formed group of NYbased companies, publishing houses, and researchers dedicated to advancing speech technology research and development.

Ladan Baghai-Ravary · Steve W. Beet

Automatic Speech Signal Analysis for Clinical Diagnosis and Assessment of Speech Disorders

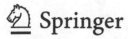 Springer

Ladan Baghai-Ravary
Phonetics Laboratory
University of Oxford
Oxford OX1 2JF
UK

Steve W. Beet
Aculab plc
Milton Keynes MK1 1PT
UK

ISSN 2191-8112   ISSN 2191-8120 (electronic)
ISBN 978-1-4614-4573-9   ISBN 978-1-4614-4574-6 (eBook)
DOI 10.1007/978-1-4614-4574-6
Springer New York Heidelberg Dordrecht London

Library of Congress Control Number: 2012941416

Printed on acid-free paper

Springer is part of Springer Science+Business Media (www.springer.com)

Preface

The diagnosis and monitoring of many common neurological conditions routinely involve acoustic analysis of the subject's speech by an expert clinician. There are two significant problems with this: one is that the analysis is time-consuming, hence expensive, and therefore often performed too infrequently, and the other is that the results of the analysis are inconsistent, depending both on the subjective opinions of the clinician and the emotional and physical state of the subject at the time the speech is sampled.

The potential advantages offered by automatic and semi-automatic speech analysis methods have been widely recognized for many years, but more recently, devices with the ability to record and process high quality audio data have become commonplace (laptop and tablet computers, smart-phones, etc.). Such devices make it even easier than before to perform frequent and informal recordings, along with at least some of the subsequent signal analysis, without any direct involvement by a speech and language therapist.

In this book, we draw on a wide range of research from laboratories around the World, and discuss the environments in which the research is performed and the apparent significance of their results. The nature of the tasks being attempted, the availability of appropriate data (both for development purposes and for evaluation), and the details of the evaluation methodology and criteria can all have a significant effect on published results. These issues are discussed and suggestions are made regarding future developments which need to be addressed to facilitate progress in the fields of automatic diagnosis and telemonitoring of disordered speech.

Despite having been an active area of research for many years, there are still many signal processing and pattern recognition techniques which have not yet been applied to disordered speech (a preliminary experiment using one such technique is described here). It seems more than likely that one or more of these could provide additional cues which are not exploited in current systems. It is hoped that the comments and discussions in this book will help to guide researchers in the development of new methods and thus improve the quality and effectiveness of diagnosis and treatment of speech-related disorders.

Contents

Chapter 1
Introduction

Abstract The focus of this book is the methods which have been proposed over the last 15–20 years for automatic analysis of speech to aid speech and language therapists and other skilled clinical practitioners in diagnosing and assessing speech disorders. This introductory chapter explains why it is now especially timely to develop new automatic methods, and summarises some of the features normally associated with disordered speech together with some aspects of current clinical practice. We also discuss some aspects of the current environment in which research, development, and evaluations of potential methods are performed, and the level of automation which may be expected in the near future. The importance of standardised testing data and procedures is critical in assessing technology in this field, so the availability of suitable testing data is discussed.

Keywords Automatic methods · Disordered speech · Remote diagnosis · Speech databases · Telemonitoring

In this text, we discuss many previously proposed methods designed to aid clinicians in the diagnosis and monitoring of neurological speech disorders such as dysphonia, dysarthria, and apraxia of speech (AOS). In particular we examine the various signal processing techniques, the statistical validity of the results presented in the literature, and the appropriateness of the methods for use "in the field"—i.e. without the need for specialised equipment, rigorously controlled recording procedures, or highly skilled personnel to interpret results.

The envisaged scenario would begin with the collection of examples of the subjects' speech, either over the phone or using portable recording devices operated by non-specialist staff, or by the subjects themselves (where practical). The recordings could then be analysed to aid diagnosis of the conditions, and subsequently regular recordings could be analysed to monitor the clients' progress and response to treatment (telemonitoring).

L. Baghai-Ravary and S. W. Beet, *Automatic Speech Signal Analysis for Clinical Diagnosis and Assessment of Speech Disorders*, SpringerBriefs in Speech Technology, DOI: 10.1007/978-1-4614-4574-6_1, © The Author(s) 2013

1.1 Progress in Remote Diagnosis and Telemonitoring

Numerous techniques for automatic evaluation of speech disorders have been proposed over the last 20 years, but the relative merits of different approaches and the relative usefulness of some aspects of the speech signal are only now becoming apparent. This book explores these issues so as to guide future research and development in this area.

Automatic diagnosis and assessment of speech pathologies has been investigated in many papers. Some recent examples include (Hawley et al. 2005) and (Maier et al. 2009). Such techniques offer the promise of a simple and cost-effective, yet objective, assessment of a range of medical conditions, which are potentially of great value to clinicians.

Currently, extended clinical tests are required to determine whether disruptions in speech development reflect a pathological condition or are momentary symptoms in long-term speech normalisation (Shriberg 1994). An automated system for collecting and performing preliminary analysis of the subject's speech has the potential to dramatically reduce the time needed to accurately diagnose or monitor speech disorders. By allowing the speech to be collected over a longer period of time, the ultimate diagnosis can also be made with a greater level of confidence.

1.2 Technological Issues

Recent years have seen widespread deployment of smart-phones and other portable devices with the ability to make good quality recordings of speech and even video, and either to process it locally or to transmit it over broadband data connections to remote systems for later analysis. This means that now, for the first time, it has become feasible (and economical) to provide frequent, regular, and objective assessments, and to provide them in a timely fashion (i.e. at short notice). This latter point is especially important in cases where the severity of the symptoms of a condition changes markedly over a short timescale.

Such technology also opens up the possibility of not just diagnosis and assessment, but also therapy being performed remotely (for some conditions at least). For example using a system such as that described in Yin et al. (2009), where the authors describe an approach to pronunciation verification for a speech therapy application.

1.3 Symptoms of Speech Impairment

Clinical diagnostic symptoms of disordered speech include hypernasality, breathiness, diplophonia, audible nasal emissions, short phrases, pitch breaks, monopitch, monoloudness, reduced loudness, slow and regular syllable "alternating motion rate" (AMR, or diadochokinesis), harshness, low pitch, slow rate, short rushes of speech and reduced stress, hypotonicity, atrophy, facial myokymia, fasciculation, occasional nasal regurgitation, dysphagia and drooling. Most (but clearly not all) of these can be analysed and graded from audio recordings of speech, and so could be utilised in telemonitoring applications.

Speech disorders can be classified in a number of ways, based on the perceived characteristics of the subject's speech. Classifications used in the literature include:

- articulatory delays, disturbed nasality (hypernasality/hyponasality), stuttering, or dysarthria (Abou-Elsaad 2010)
- organic or non-organic, neurological or non-neurological, benign or malignant, and hyperfunctional dysphonia or hypofunctional dysphonia, phononeurosis or dysodia (Pützer and Koreman 1997).

Further, each of these categories of disorder can be further sub-divided (Duffy 2011), based on particular combinations of symptoms, as identified by the clinician. For example, dysarthria can be classed as ataxic, spastic, flaccid, hypokinetic, hyperkinetic or unilateral upper motor neuron, or a mixture of these. Each such form of dysarthria is associated with a different neurological locus, and may exhibit different symptoms as a result.

Thus, there are a very large number of possible detailed diagnoses of any suspected speech disorder, and differentiating between many of them relies on combinations of symptoms, some of which are not available in simple audio recordings. As such, for the foreseeable future, a detailed diagnosis will always require analysis by an expert clinician.

Nonetheless, many researchers have realised that they could provide an automatic system to aid the clinician in reaching their diagnosis, reducing the time they would need to spend listening to each individual patient, and increasing the reliability of the result.

Furthermore, the objectivity and repeatability of an automatic analysis can be enhanced by integrating statistics of the patient's speech collected over many hours, or even choosing the time for the recording to coincide with a particular time of day, or with the severity of the symptoms, as perceived by the subjects themselves.

1.4 Diagnosis and Assessment

Traditionally diagnosis can involve neurological, radiological, psychological, and perceptual (acoustic) assessment methods. Cummings (2008) provides a very thorough and informed description of both the clinical aspects of speech disorders, and the level of uncertainty and even controversy which surrounds their diagnosis and treatment.

Relevant standardised perceptual tests include the Boston Diagnostic Aphasia Examination (BDAE), the Western Aphasia Battery, the Buffalo III Voice Profile, the Apraxia Battery for Adults, and the Frenchay Dysarthria Assessment (FDA).

These typically involve grading various aspects of the subject's speech on a 4 or 5-point scale.

Biases and inconsistencies in perceptual judgment have been well documented (Tversky 1969), and, as was investigated in Mehta and Hillman (2008), there can be significant differences between assessments, even when performed by expert clinicians. In some cases, this can be due to short-term changes in the severity or character of the symptoms of the patient, but there is also a level of inconsistency in any given clinician's interpretation of the symptoms, and a somewhat larger inconsistency between one clinician and another.

It has been shown (Koreman and Pützer 2003) that in clinical practice, the differences between individual clinicians are not as important as might be expected, however: each clinician learns to interpret their own assessment scales and they usually go on to arrive at a similar diagnosis. Thus, provided the same clinician assesses the subject's speech, as makes the ultimate diagnosis, the end result will usually be the same.

Nonetheless, for the scenario being considered here, it should not be expected that an algorithm which closely reproduces any specific clinician's assessment of voice quality will necessarily allow another clinician to perform accurate diagnosis; at least, not without a lengthy training or acclimatisation procedure, where the clinician can learn to interpret the automatic assessments appropriately.

1.5 Performance Evaluation of Algorithms and Systems

Some researchers have suggested that any automatic diagnostic tool should be strongly correlated with standard acoustic/perceptual measures if it is to be of clinical value. This appears to be more of an assumption than a demonstrable fact. Nonetheless, there are a number of reports where a correlation between human assessments, with automatically calculated estimates of traditional clinical speech characteristics, has been used to infer the superiority of one method over another.

If a new method of automatic assessment is to be evaluated, it is only of marginal interest to demonstrate a correlation with human assessments of acoustic measures such as breathiness, and even intelligibility. It is only once an automatic algorithm has been fully developed (or an expert clinician fully trained) to differentiate between conditions using those measures, that they can be optimised or compared with any alternatives.

Another issue that has plagued this field is the scarcity of sufficiently comprehensive databases of speech recordings. For many years there has been only one publicly available database of substantial size, the Massachusetts Eye and Ear Infirmary (MEEI) database, which forms part of the Disordered Voice Database and Program from KayPENTAX®. This contains two samples of speech from each of 53 normal and 657 pathological speakers. The database includes the first 12 s of each speaker speaking a standard text, "The Rainbow Passage" (Fairbanks 1960), and also a sustained phonation of the phoneme /a/ (as in "father"). This database is marketed primarily as a training resource to familiarise clinicians with the interpretation of the parameters calculated by the MDVP™ software. Nonetheless, it is widely used in the development and performance evaluation of new algorithms, largely because of its size and wide availability.[1]

Other smaller databases were recorded around the same time, including the Nemours database of 11 male dysarthric speakers (Menéndez-Pidal et al. 1996) and the Whitaker database of North American English subjects with cerebral palsy (Deller et al. 1993).

Apart from these, researchers associated with different institutions have often collected their own data, and it appears from their descriptions in the literature that some of these databases are of a reasonable size, and often more specialised, giving a more thorough characterisation of a specific speech disorder for the task at hand. Historically, most of this data has not been made available outside the respective institutions. This has meant that the only meaningful way for researchers outside such institutions to assess or compare proposed systems, has been to evaluate them using the MEEI data.

In more recent years, additional data has started to become more freely available, most notably the Alborada-I3A database for Spanish children's speech (Saz et al. 2010) and another, commonly referred to as the "Universal Access" database (Kim et al. 2008), again concentrating on North American dysarthric speakers with cerebral palsy. This latter database may prove to be of greater significance to some researchers because it includes simultaneous recordings from eight separate microphones and a video camera, allowing for the study of both non-acoustical parameters, and of the effect of (some) variations in the acoustic environment.

Possibly because of the lack of diversity in the recording conditions of the previously available data, literature in this area has been largely theoretical in nature, and only occasionally explored the effects of "real-world" factors on the data being analysed. Most databases of disordered speech have been recorded with as much control of the recording environment as possible—far more rigorously than would be possible "in the field".

As well as the lack of diversity in recording conditions, large quantities of data are only available for a few languages—mostly North American English, with smaller datasets in Spanish, non-American variants of English and one or two other languages such as Korean.

---

[1] KayPENTAX® Disordered Voice Database and Program, Model 4337 includes their Multi-Dimensional Voice Program (MDVP™) and the Computerized Speech Lab (CSL™)/Multi-Speech™ software. Further information can be found on their web site (http://www.kaypentax.com/).

References

Abou-Elsaad T (2010) Auditory perceptual assessment of voice and speech disorders. In: Presentation at the 28th Alexandria international congress (Comb ORL). http://alexorl.com/page/The28thAlexandriaInternationalCongress(Combined%20ORL). Accessed 16 Feb 2012

Cummings L (2008) Clinical linguistics. Edinburgh University Press Ltd, Edinburgh. ISBN 978 0 7486 2077 7

Deller JR, Liu MS, Ferrier LJ, Robichaud P (1993) The Whitaker database of dysarthric (cerebral palsy) speech. J Acoust Soc Am 93(6):3516–3518. doi:10.1121/1.405684

Duffy JR (2011) Differential diagnosis among the dysarthrias—the rules of the game. In: Presentation at the Texas speech-language-hearing association 2011 Convention. http://www.txsha.org/convention/handouts2011.aspx. Accessed 16 Feb 2012

Fairbanks G (1960) Voice and articulation drillbook, 2nd edn. Harper & Row, New York, pp 124–139

Hawley MS, Green PD, Enderby P, Cunningham SP, Moore RK (2005) Speech technology for e-inclusion of people with physical disabilities and disordered speech. In Proceedings of INTERSPEECH-2005, pp 445–448

Kim H, Hasegawa-Johnson M, Perlman A, Gunderson J, Huang T, Watkin K, Frame S (2008) Dysarthric speech database for universal access research. In Proceedings of INTERSPEECH-2008, pp 1741–1744

Koreman J, Pützer M (2003) The usability of perceptual ratings of voice quality. In: Proceedings of 6th international conference: advances in quantitative laryngology, voice and speech research (AQL 2003)

Maier A, Haderlein T, Eysholdt U, Rosanowski F, Batliner A, Schuster M, Nöth E (2009) PEAKS—a system for the automatic evaluation of voice and speech disorders. Speech Commun 51(5):425–437. doi:10.1016/j.specom.2009.01.004

Mehta DD, Hillman RE (2008) Voice assessment: updates on perceptual, acoustic, aerodynamic, and endoscopic imaging methods. Curr Opin Otolaryngol Head Neck Surg 16(3):211–215. doi:10.1097/MOO.0b013e3282fe96ce

Menéndez-Pidal X, Polikoff JB, Peters SM, Leonzio JE, Bunnell HT (1996) The Nemours database of dysarthric speech. In: Proceedings of 4th international conference on spoken language processing (ICSLP), vol 3, pp 1962–1965. doi:10.1109/ICSLP.1996.608020

Pützer M, Koreman J (1997) A German database of patterns of pathological vocal fold vibration. PHONUS 3:143–153

Saz O, Lleida E, Vaquero C, Rodríguez WR (2010) The Alborada-I3A corpus of disordered speech. In: Proceedings of language resources and evaluation conference LREC-2010, pp 2814–2819

Shriberg LD (1994) Five subtypes of developmental phonological disorders. Clinics in Commun Disord 4:38–53

Tversky A (1969) Intransitivity of preferences. Psychol Rev 76:31–48. doi:10.1037/h0026750

Yin S-C, Rose R, Saz O, Lleida E (2009) A study of pronunciation verification in a speech therapy application. In Proceedings of IEEE international conference on acoustics, speech, and signal processing ICASSP-2009, pp 4609–4612

Chapter 2
Speech Production and Perception

Abstract Certain specific characteristics of speech are known to be particularly useful in diagnosing speech disorders by acoustic (perceptual) and instrumental methods. The most widely cited of these are described in this chapter, along with some comments as to their suitability for use in automated systems. Some of these features can be characterised by relatively simple signal processing operations, while others would ideally require a realistic model of the higher levels of neurological processing, including cognition. It is observed that even experts who come to the same ultimate decision regarding diagnosis, often differ in their assessment of individual speech characteristics. The difficulties of quantifying prosody and accurately identifying pitch epochs are highlighted, because of their importance in human perception of speech disorders.

Keywords Characteristics of disordered speech · Objective assessment of vocal characteristics · Precision of articulation · Subjectivity of perception

The higher levels of neural processing involved in both speech production and speech perception are still only partially understood. There is even some degree of controversy regarding the detailed mechanical functioning of the peripheral auditory system (Shera and Olson 2011), despite having been the subject of research for many years.

According to Duffy (2000), "speech is the most complex of innately acquired human motor skills, an activity characterised in normal adults by the production of about 14 distinguishable sounds per second through the coordinated actions of about 100 muscles innervated by multiple cranial and spinal nerves". Furthermore, speech production involves great temporal precision (in the region of 10 ms), while some parts of the peripheral auditory system have been found to exhibit an even greater resolution—in the region of 10 μs (Fuchs 2005).

The complexity of these processes, and the fine temporal resolution they utilise makes precise diagnosis of the location of neural damage extremely difficult, and

L. Baghai-Ravary and S. W. Beet, *Automatic Speech Signal Analysis for Clinical Diagnosis and Assessment of Speech Disorders*, SpringerBriefs in Speech Technology, DOI: 10.1007/978-1-4614-4574-6_2, © The Author(s) 2013

only some of the features proposed for use in diagnostic aids should be expected to yield useful and reliable information.

Masaki (2010) provides a thorough and well thought-out description of the field and discusses development of the voice production structures. She mentions that some are not fully developed, even until the age of 25, so it should be borne in mind that voice production is not a stable and fixed process, even for one individual, and the effect of some pathologies on the voice will be more or less profound at different stages of vocal development.

2.1 Articulation

At the core of the definition of the term "dysarthria", is mis-articulation of the sounds in spoken words. It can manifest itself in all aspects of speech production: phonation, resonance, articulation and respiration. As such, analysis of the accuracy of articulation is clearly important to diagnosis and telemonitoring.

The accuracy of articulation can be affected by many factors—both neurological (as in cerebral palsy, for example, where the precision, speed and variety of the sounds is often restricted) and physical (due to factors such as the health of the muscles used to produce the sounds). The situation is somewhat complicated since long-term neurological conditions can adversely affect physical attributes such as muscle tonicity. In fluent speech, articulation can be abnormally restricted (if the muscles are hypertonic, as in spastic cerebral palsy) or abnormally large (if they are hypotonic). The various articulators can be affected to different degrees depending on the specific condition. Articulation can also be affected by physical or neurological damage in the mechanisms associated with speech production. Even disturbances affecting the subject's perception of their own speech can cause abnormal articulation.

Whenever articulation is disturbed, it generally becomes more difficult to understand the speech, so a speech and language therapist will generally grade the intelligibility (see below) as part of the assessment. A more detailed analysis of the exact form of the disturbance can be very time-consuming.

2.2 Phonation

The term "phonation" refers to periodic modulations of the air pressure from the lungs by the opening and closing of the vocal folds. There are a number of causes of atypical phonation, both physical and neurological in origin.

Phonation can become irregular in terms of pitch ("jitter"), or in terms of amplitude ("shimmer"), or it can be polluted with aperiodic noise, caused by turbulence around a constriction in the airway, for example. The presence of aperiodic noise is conventionally quantified via the harmonic-to-noise ratio, HNR. It is also very common for the maximum duration of sustained phonation to be restricted in pathological speech. All of these factors are routinely assessed using computerised analysis of the speech waveform, although they can only be evaluated accurately and repeatably from sustained vowel phonations.

For the purposes of assessing phonation, it is common to analyse sustained production of the /a/ vowel (/a/ as in "father"), and indeed for automatic systems, it has been shown that this specific vowel offers noticeably better accuracy than others (Henríquez et al. 2009).

2.3 Voicing

A number of structures can be utilised for the production of the acoustic pressure wave that excites the resonances of the vocal tract. This excitation signal can be one or more of periodic, transient, or stochastic (fricative) in nature. Any abnormality can be heard in the resulting speech, and the type of voicing can usually be identified quite reliably by automatic methods.

A number of speech disorders can manifest themselves as this type of abnormality. For example, phonation may be present during what should be fricative sounds, or there may be errors which effectively realise a voiced stop as unvoiced, or vice versa.

2.4 Resonance

When voiced speech is produced, energy may be coupled into the nasal cavity, introducing an additional resonance and anti-resonance into the overall vocal tract response. Perceptual assessments of speech quality attempt to quantify the effectiveness of the nasal coupling by gauging the degree of "nasal resonance".

Some tests additionally assess the "oral resonance" of the speech, which is a measure of how far "back in the throat" the voice is perceived as being.

Both oral and nasal resonance is usually assessed from read passages containing both nasal and non-nasal sounds. The presence or absence of nasal resonance can be determined quite easily, especially in context (the onset of nasal sounds is clearly visible in a spectrogram, for example) but oral resonance is difficult to quantify precisely, and thus difficult to analyse automatically.

2.5 Prosody

The intonation, stress, and rhythm of speech, i.e. the prosody, contains a disproportionate amount of high-level non-verbal information, much of which is used socially, and as such, is adversely affected in a number of neurological conditions, especially those which affect social interaction. Prosody is also readily disrupted by problems of respiration. Both the pitch and the intensity of the speech can become more difficult to control if the supply of air to the vocal folds is too low or too variable.

In terms of the analysis of prosody, van Santen et al. (2009) suggests that the data produced by commercial software such as the KayPENTAX® Multi-Dimensional Voice Program, MDVP™, is only marginally relevant to prosody, even though prosody is generally believed to be key in perceptual/acoustic assessment of disorders. This is because the phonetician's concept of prosody is defined at a more abstract level, concerned with concepts such as "stress", "intonation" and "rhythm", which can be assessed in terms of "naturalness" and other perceived characteristics, but which cannot be defined precisely via mathematical equations.

The data provided by automatic systems can only represent statistics of the signal, either integrated over a varied example of speech (e.g. the range and stability of pitch during a sentence), or evaluated independently over individual speech sounds (jitter or shimmer measured during sustained phonation, voice-onset-time (VOT) for stop consonants, etc.).

van Santen et al. (2009) goes on to quote others saying that dialect-differences can be as large as language-differences in prosody, and accents can cause problems for both human and automatic assessment. They also discuss the advantages human assessment can offer because of the ability to adapt to accent, voice quality, speaking style, etc.

It can be inferred from Kent (1996) that human assessment cannot be relied on to provide a benchmark for the development of automatic prosodic analysis: "the acoustic correlates of prosody are perceptually much too complex to be fully categorized into items by humans—they cannot be reliably judged by humans who have subjective opinions". That is to say that there is currently no way to characterise the subtleties of prosody in a tractable mathematical form.

Nonetheless, a number of useful mathematical features related to prosody have been defined, (e.g. Pentland 2007; Schuller et al. 2007), and they can identify at least some gross abnormalities in prosody. Despite such progress in defining a wide set of prosodic features, there is still no clear consensus as to the most effective or efficient features (Ringeval et al. 2010).

2.6 Intelligibility

For many conditions, where a simple measure of its severity is required to monitor response to treatment, for example, a perceptual assessment of intelligibility can be used.

As long as the sounds being produced can be controlled as part of the assessment protocol, intelligibility can be assessed acoustically, although there is evidence that different listeners may produce noticeably different evaluations (McHenry 2011). Indeed in (Ziegler and Zierdt 2008) it was found to be necessary to average the results of 2 or 3 different listeners in order to produce a reliable correlation between manual and automatic measures, recorded on a simple percentage scale. When assessment is to be performed by a single listener, a graded assessment is more appropriate (on a 4 or 5 point scale, for example).

References

Duffy JR (2000) Motor speech disorders: clues to neurologic diagnosis. In: Adler CH, Ahlskog JE (eds) Parkinson's disease and movement disorders: diagnosis and treatment guidelines for the practicing physician. Humana Press, Totowa, pp 35–53

Fuchs PA (2005) Time and intensity coding at the hair cell's ribbon synapse. J Physiol 566(1):7–12

Henríquez P, Alonso JB, Ferrer MA, Travieso CM, Godino-Llorente JI, Díaz-de-María F (2009) Characterization of healthy and pathological voice through measures based on nonlinear dynamics. IEEE Trans Audio Speech Lang Process 17(6):1186–1195

Kent RD (1996) Hearing and believing: some limits to the auditory-perceptual assessment of speech and voice disorders. Am J Speech-Lang Pathol 5(3):7–23

Masaki A (2010) Optimizing acoustic and perceptual assessment of voice quality in children with vocal nodules. PhD thesis, Harvard-MIT Health Sciences and Technology

McHenry M (2011) An exploration of listener variability in intelligibility judgments. Am J Speech-Lang Pathol 20:119–123. doi:10.1044/1058-0360(2010/10-0059

Pentland A (2007) Social signal processing. IEEE Signal Process Mag 24(4):108–111

Ringeval F, Demouy J, Szaszák G, Chetouani M, Robel L, Xavier J, Cohen D, Plaza M (2010) Automatic intonation recognition for the prosodic assessment of language-impaired children. IEEE Trans Audio Speech Lang Process 19(5):1328–1342. doi:10.1109/TASL.2010.2090147

Schuller B, Batliner A, Seppi D, Steidl S, Vogt T, Wagner J, Devillers L, Vidrascu L, Amir N, Kessous L, Aharonson V (2007) The relevance of feature type for the automatic classification of emotional user states: low level descriptors and functionals. In: Proceedings of INTERSPEECH-2007, pp 2253–2256

Shera CA, Olson ES (eds) (2011) What fire is in mine ears: progress in auditory biomechanics. In: Proceedings of 11th international mechanics of hearing workshop. American Institute of Physics, Melville

van Santen JPH, Prud'hommeaux ET, Black LM (2009) Automated assessment of prosody production. Speech Commun 51(11):1082–1097. doi:10.1016/j.specom.2009.04.007

Ziegler W, Zierdt A (2008) Telediagnostic assessment of intelligibility in dysarthria: a pilot investigation of MVP-online. J Commun Disord 41(6):553–577

Chapter 3
Acoustic Effects of Speech Impairment

Abstract Some of the most common forms of speech impairment are summarised here, in terms of their main distinctive acoustic and temporal characteristics (rhythm, intonation, etc.). Where they offer significant advantages, we also mention some non-acoustic methods for assessment and diagnosis. The speech disorders considered in this book are neurological in origin: primarily dysphonia, dysprosody, dysarthria and apraxia of speech, but we also mention some considerations relevant to the diagnosis of stuttering, Parkinson's disease and even schizophrenia. It is suggested that the tasks of assessing severity of a condition, and of differential diagnosis, need not use the same acoustic features, and indeed there may be significant advantages in using complementary features and procedures for the two tasks.

Keywords Acoustic perceptual assessment · Jitter · Neurological speech impairments · Shimmer · Standard scales and procedures

There are many aspects of speech which can be assessed acoustically, although there is no single procedure which is appropriate to every case. For example, Masaki (2010) points out that the Consensus Auditory Perceptual Evaluation of Voice (CAPE-V) test requires reading six sentences, and so is not suitable for pre-literate children. The CAPE-V protocol involves scores for overall severity, roughness, breathiness, strain, pitch and loudness. She goes on to describe a paediatric version of CAPE-V which gives better correlation between human scorers, suggesting that its results should be more reliable.

Middag et al. (2009) point out that the correlation between intelligibility (measured on the 7-point Likert scale) and automatic speech recognition (ASR) accuracy quoted in many papers, only holds for specific pathologies.

Similarly, other traditional measures of a condition's severity are only useful for a limited range of conditions. Such condition-specific measures can nonetheless be useful since they can provide discrimination between conditions. That is to

L. Baghai-Ravary and S. W. Beet, *Automatic Speech Signal Analysis for Clinical Diagnosis and Assessment of Speech Disorders*, SpringerBriefs in Speech Technology, DOI: 10.1007/978-1-4614-4574-6_3, © The Author(s) 2013

say, that discrimination *between* conditions often requires quite different forms of analysis from those used to assess the *severity* of the condition. To gain an insight into which features are most useful for these two distinct tasks, the acoustic effects of the different classes of speech disorder must be considered.

In theory at least, there is no reason why a method which is totally unrelated to perceptual interpretation of speech sounds, should not yield just as much, or an even greater, ability to discriminate between different forms of speech disorder.

3.1 Dysphonia

Dysphonia is a term for disorders of phonation, as opposed to dysarthria, which is an impairment of the ability to produce spoken words. Dysphonia may be perceived as roughness due to irregular movement of the glottis.

Although dysphonia can be measured using a variety of methods that visualise the pattern of vibration of the vocal folds (e.g. laryngeal stroboscopy), acoustic examination is also commonplace. Subjective measurement of the severity of dysphonia may be carried out by trained clinical staff using (for example) the GRBAS (grade, roughness, breathiness, asthenia, strain) scale or the Oates Perceptual Profile. Objective measurement of the severity of dysphonia typically requires signal processing algorithms applied to acoustic and/or electro-glottograph recordings.

Features commonly calculated include jitter, shimmer and noise-to-harmonics ratio (NHR). These features require an accurate pitch estimate with a high temporal resolution, which is difficult for real-world signals, especially when the jitter or shimmer is severe. Many pitch tracking algorithms rely on linear or non-linear smoothing of local pitch estimates, which often vary markedly from one analysis epoch to the next. Recent advances in signal processing theory have led to more robust algorithms, but there is still much room for improvement.

3.2 Dysprosody

Dysprosody is characterised by alterations in intensity, segmental timing, rhythm, cadence, and intonation of words. The changes to the duration, fundamental frequency, and the syllable intensity, deprive an individual's speech of its personal characteristics. The cause of dysprosody is usually associated with neurological pathologies such as vascular accidents in the brain (stroke), cranio-encephalic trauma, and brain tumours.

In some ways, dysarthria (see below) can manifest itself much like a combination of dysphonia and dysprosody, although dysprosody is less commonly diagnosed than either dysphonia or dysarthria.

van Santen et al. (2009) tried to distinguish between effects using prosodic minimal pairs and found automatic methods were mostly as good as humans at assessing severity of condition. They used many different approaches to improving performance—constraining the elicitation procedure to minimise non-pathology-related variations, using robust signal analyses, weighted combinations of features, limiting age range to 4–8 years, and concentrating on autism spectrum disorder (ASD). Some of the elicitation methods were probably difficult for patients with severe conditions, but they also restricted the IQ range to greater than 70, which should ameliorate the problem somewhat. They also excluded a range of neurological conditions (such as cerebral palsy, brain lesions, etc.) and restricted the normal speakers to those with no significant familial speech/language disorders. They used assessments by a set of clinicians, and another set of naïve listeners.

3.3 Dysarthria

Dysarthria can be caused by a weakness or paralysis of speech muscles resulting from neural damage, leading to imprecise, slow and/or distorted verbal communications. Dysarthria is often caused by strokes, Parkinson's disease, motor neurone disease, head or neck injuries, surgical accident, or cerebral palsy.

Portnoy and Aronson (1982) found a slower and more variable syllable rate in adult subjects with spastic dysarthria. This observation is typical of reported characteristics of dysarthric speech: the disorder is at a higher level than simple dysphonia—it is not simply the instantaneous acoustic characteristics of the speech which are affected, but the durational structure and the dynamics of the speech which are abnormal.

Dysarthria is nonetheless typically characterized by slow, weak, imprecise and uncoordinated articulatory movements (Yorkston et al. 1999), brought about by paralysis or poor co-ordination of some part of the speech mechanism (larynx, lips, tongue, palate and jaw). Thus we would expect an unusually uniform level of 'dynamics' in dysarthric speech, with phoneme transitions being less abrupt than normal, and periods of steady phonation being less stable.

3.4 Apraxia of Speech

Apraxia of speech manifests itself at a higher level still. Subjects suffering from apraxia of speech (AOS) may have varying rates, rhythms and stresses to their speech. Their speech may be perceived as having an unusual accent or cadence. They may also have difficulties with non-speech language-related tasks.

Apraxia of speech may be acquired (e.g. following a stroke) or developmental, and involves inconsistencies in the production of speech sounds, often resulting in a re-ordering of the phonemes within a word. The more effort a speaker puts into the production of the words, the more likely they are to be incorrect. They may say a word correctly, but then mispronounce it a short time later.

Acquired apraxia of speech is mostly present in adults and is often the result of injury to the part of the brain that controls language use, commonly as the result of a stroke. Developmental apraxia of speech occurs mainly in children and is often present from birth.

According to Ogar et al. (2005), apraxia of speech "… is often the first symptom of neurodegenerative diseases, such as primary progressive aphasia and corticobasal degeneration". Also "… symptoms associated with AOS often co-occur or overlap with those caused by neuromuscular deficits indicative of the dysarthrias and the linguistic errors associated with aphasia." but, "When diagnosing AOS, it is important to distinguish the disorder from Broca's aphasia, conduction aphasia and dysarthria …" because of its importance as an early clinical indicator of progressive neurologic disease.

Apraxia of speech was studied in Shriberg et al. (2004), which examined parameters derived from (i) durations of speech and pauses and (ii) vowel duration, pitch and amplitude, although these parameters would also be expected to be indicative of dysarthric speech. As such, these parameters could be useful for monitoring progress during therapy, but are less likely to be good discriminative indicators.

Cera and Ortiz (2010) states "… patients with apraxia of speech produce not only phonetic errors (e.g. distortions) but also phonemic errors (e.g. substitutions, deletions, insertions, reduplications, metatheses, etc.)". This paper is based on Brazilian Portuguese, using part of the "Boston Diagnostic Aphasia Examination", analysing phonological features based on the distinctive features model proposed in Chomsky and Halle (1968) and the Consonant Segments Matrix for the Portuguese language including sonorant, syllabic, consonantal, continuant, strident, delayed release, nasal, lateral, anterior, coronal, high, low, posterior and voiced classes. The patients had suffered strokes, and most had different types of aphasia and apraxia. They found the most affected features to be voiced, continuant, high, low, anterior, coronal and posterior, as opposed to coronal, continuant, anterior, strident, posterior, high and voiced, as found in a previous study of aphasics, which had been specific to Portuguese. They cite a number of studies which suggest the biggest indicator of apraxic speech is devoicing of voiced phonemes. Unsurprisingly they observed that "the number of errors increases with complexity of motor adjustment needed for articulation".

Thoonen (1998) used "Speech Lab" to analyse pitch (Reetz 1989), syllable duration, etc. He looked at a number of parameters, and concluded that just two (mean monosyllabic repetition rate and maximum phonation duration) were enough to differentiate between dysarthria, developmental apraxia of speech, and a set of normal controls. The other parameters he considered were maximum fricative duration, variability in repetition rate, the number of attempts needed to correctly produce a tri-syllabic sequence, mean tri-syllabic repetition rate, the ratio of mean tri-syllabic repetition rate to mean monosyllabic repetition rate.

The use of syllable-level (or greater) measures appears to be the key to differentiation between apraxia of speech and the lower-level disorders, dysarthria and dysphonia.

3.5 Aphasia

Aphasia is a more linguistic or cognitively focussed disorder which results in an impaired ability to produce or comprehend language, whether written or spoken. It can occur in combination with other communication difficulties. Many different types of aphasias exist, all with particular signs and symptoms.

Bhogal et al. (2003) points out that the intensity of any speech therapy is important, even in aphasic patients. Difficulty recalling words or names is the most long-lasting symptom of aphasia. For both aphasia, and stuttering (below) there is little indication in the acoustic signal as to the nature of the disorder. A transcription of the words and/or phonemes articulated by the subject is needed to identify the condition.

3.6 Stuttering

Davis et al. (2000) divided subjects into stutterers who responded to treatment, those who didn't, and those who were suspected stutterers but may have been misdiagnosed. Their review of the diagnosis of stuttering suggests that speech measures alone are wholly insufficient for reliable diagnosis. Indeed, scores based on recorded speech are only one out of ten key factors in differentiating stuttering from other disorders or "normal non-fluencies". Even when estimating the prognosis for recovery, the family history and the child's attitude are at least as important as any actual measurements of the child's speech.

The most pertinent aspects of the speech signal appear to be abnormal prolongation, and articulation errors. However there is still a lack of consensus regarding exactly how these features should be used in diagnosis.

An additional factor has inhibited the use of speech measures with respect to stuttering. That is the marked changes in symptoms which are observed as a result of the subject's emotional state, their familiarity with their environment, etc. This effect is unusually marked in the case of stuttering. Given that this factor is widely acknowledged, it is surprisingly common for diagnosis to be performed on the basis of a single recording. Generally, that recording will have been made in a clinical setting where the unknown level of stress or unfamiliarity of the patient, will add an additional uncontrolled factor to the assessment, reducing the diagnostic value of any measures of the subject's speech.

3.7 Parkinson's Disease

Speech-related symptoms of Parkinson's disease include reduced volume (hypophonia), reduced pitch range, and dysarthria. Additionally there can be language problems that can further affect the subject's speech. For example, maximum repetition rates have been used for assessment of cerebral palsy, Parkinsonism and functional articulation disorders, including lisping, since as early as 1972 (Fletcher 1972). Assessment, even via such straightforward parameters as these, and by an experienced clinician, can take 20–30 min, not counting the time for recording. There have been a significant number of attempts to detect/diagnose/assess Parkinson's disease on the basis of speech recordings, some of which are discussed later in this book.

3.8 Schizophrenia

Schizophrenia is more often thought of as a cognitive disorder, with disorganised and delusional thought processes, hallucinations, apathy and social isolation as common symptoms. However, Cummings (2008) points out that there are also a number of linguistic and vocal symptoms which could be exploited in telemonitoring applications. In particular, she notes that "affective flattening, … (and disruption of) … phonology, morphology, syntax, semantics, and pragmatics" are all correlated with schizophrenia.

Affective flattening and disruptions to phonology could potentially be detected with current technologies, although the position with regard to the other "disruptions" is less clear-cut. To the best of the authors' knowledge, there have been no publications to date which have attempted to automate the detection or assessment of schizophrenia on the basis of speech recordings.

References

Bhogal SK, Teasell R, Speechley M (2003) Intensity of aphasia therapy, impact on recovery. Stroke 34:987–993. doi:10.1161/01.str.0000062343.64383.d0

Cera ML, Ortiz KZ (2010) Phonological analysis of substitution errors of patients with apraxia of speech. Dementia Neuropsychol 4(1):58–62

Chomsky N, Halle M (1968) The sound pattern of english. Harper & Row, New York

Cummings L (2008) Clinical linguistics. Edinburgh University Press Ltd, Edinburgh. ISBN 978 0 7486 2077 7

Davis S, Howell P, Rustin L (2000) A multivariate approach to diagnosis and prediction of therapy outcome with children who stutter; the social status of the child who stutters. In: Baker KL, Rustin L, Cook F (eds) Proceedings of fifth oxford dysfluency conference, pp 32–41

Fletcher SG (1972) Time-by-count measurement of diadochokinetic syllable rate. J Speech Hearing Res 15:763–770

Masaki A (2010) Optimizing acoustic and perceptual assessment of voice quality in children with vocal nodules. PhD thesis, Harvard-MIT Health Sciences and Technology

Middag C, Martens J-P, van Nuffelen G, de Bodt M (2009) Automated intelligibility assessment of pathological speech using phonological features. EURASIP J Adv Signal Process. doi:10.1155/2009/629030

Ogar J, Slama H, Dronkers N, Amici S, Gorno-Tempini ML (2005) Apraxia of speech: an overview. Neurocase 11(6):427–432

Portnoy RA, Aronson AE (1982) Diadochokinetic syllable rate and regularity in normal and in spastic and ataxic dysarthric subjects. J Speech Hearing Disorders 47:324–328

Reetz H (1989) A fast expert program for pitch extraction. Proc Eurospeech 1:476–479 van Santen JPH, Prud'hommeaux ET, Black LM (2009) Automated assessment of prosody production. Speech Commun 51(11):1082–1097. doi:10.1016/j.specom.2009.04.007

Shriberg LD, Hosom J-P, Green JR (2004) Diagnostic assessment of childhood apraxia of speech using automatic speech recognition (ASR) systems. J Med Speech Lang Pathol 12(4):167–171

Thoonen GHJ (1998) Developmental apraxia of speech in children—quantitative assessment of speech characteristics. Thesis, University of Nijmegen. ISBN 90-9011330-4

Yorkston KM, Beukelman DR, Strand EA, Bell KR (1999) Management of motor speech disorders in children and adults, 2nd edn. PRO-ED, Austin

Chapter 4
Technology and Implementation

Abstract The aim of this chapter is to highlight relevant technical factors and limitations affecting collection and interpretation of speech signals. We concentrate on the typical corruption or distortion of the speech signal which is encountered in the real world, and where possible, we include an indication of how important these effects can be. Transmission and encoding of speech signals in mobile phone networks and the internet is almost invariably lossy, and this has an acute effect on the accuracy of speech recognition systems. Published research has also shown a comparable effect on the accuracy of dysphonia/dysarthria detection. The relationship between some specific aspects of the data collection process and the validity of assessments of new techniques, is discussed. The current absence of a realistic database of remotely collected speech samples is highlighted, and adherence to standardised methods and datasets is shown to be crucial to the evaluation of new algorithms. Methods for combining multiple features into a single result are frequently required, and these too are discussed in this chapter.

Keywords Databases of disordered speech · Recording procedures · Signal corruption and data loss · Speech signal processing · Speech analysis software

The technology most often used by specialist clinicians and researchers in established groups has been based around the KayPENTAX® CSL™ family of systems. For many years these hardware/software systems have provided the 'gold standard' for clinical speech analysis. They are capable of analysing speech signals with very high fidelity and calculating a multitude of acoustic characteristics to aid in diagnosis.

These systems are often used as a benchmark in assessing novel algorithms. For example, (Bakker et al. 1993) constructed a custom computer system for automated measurement of repetition rate and durational variability and revealed strong concurrent validity with reference to a carefully conducted non-automated

L. Baghai-Ravary and S. W. Beet, *Automatic Speech Signal Analysis for Clinical Diagnosis and Assessment of Speech Disorders*, SpringerBriefs in Speech Technology, DOI: 10.1007/978-1-4614-4574-6_4, © The Author(s) 2013

analysis employing the commercial system, CSL^{TM} (KayPENTAX$^{®}$, Model 4300).

There are a number of other software packages which are frequently used as benchmarks for evaluating new algorithms. Commercial software for clinical voice analysis includes "Dr Speech", as well as the MDVP^{TM} software, mentioned previously. Like MDVP^{TM}, "Dr Speech" calculates many parameters: habitual F0, jitter, shimmer, F0 tremor, F0 statistics (mean, standard deviation, maximum and minimum), amplitude tremor, and a number of others.[1]

One other piece of software, not normally used by clinicians, but very useful for research into computer analysis of speech pathology, is Praat (Boersma and Weenink 2009). A number of researchers have also used programs such as the CSLU toolkit (Sutton et al. 1998) for prompting and recording, the Snack toolkit (Sjölander 2004) to obtain pitch (based on an algorithm used originally in the Entropic Speech Processing System[2]), and other de-facto standard software (HTK,[3] CMUSphinx,[4] WaveSurfer,[5] etc.).

4.1 Recording and Data Collection

As mentioned in Chap.1, most databases used during the development of automatic diagnostic and assessment methods have been recorded under tightly controlled conditions, by personnel experienced in such recording. This is highly desirable for any database used to develop or train an automatic speech system, but it cannot easily provide a realistic assessment of the performance which could be expected in a remote diagnosis or telemonitoring application.

There are also problems, even with well-controlled databases: sometimes due to the practicalities of recording in a clinical setting, and sometimes because of the design of the database, if it was not originally intended for use in training or evaluating automatic systems.

In particular, it is common for recordings of disordered speech to have been collected with different equipment, a different configuration, or in a different environment, from the non-disordered speech. There can also be differences in the age, gender, or other distributions of disordered and non-disordered speakers. In

---

[1] For a complete description of the Dr Speech software and the parameters it calculates, see the company's official web site: http://www.drspeech.com/

[2] ESPS is no longer commercially available, but the source code can be found at KTH, Stockholm: http://www.speech.kth.se/software/#esps

[3] HTK is available from Cambridge University Engineering Department, through http://htk.eng.cam.ac.uk/

[4] CMUSphinx is an open-source toolkit for speech recognition, developed by Carnegie Mellon University, and available via http://cmusphinx.org/

[5] WaveSurfer is an open-source tool for sound visualization and manipulation developed at KTH Stockholm: http://www.speech.kth.se/wavesurfer/.

the case of the MEEI database, for example, if age and gender distributions are to be matched between normal and pathological speakers, the majority of the disordered speech must be discarded. Typically only around 175 disordered speakers can be included out of more than 650 in the complete MEEI database.

In tele-monitoring applications, there will be many factors that can cause automatic systems serious problems. Some are due to environmental and human factors (misinterpretation of, or inability to follow, the recording protocol laid down by the designer, recovery after an error, reaction to external stimuli, background noise, etc.). Others are due to technical issues (handling noise if the recording device is hand-held, electrical noise and distortion, modification of the data by transmission via the lossy codecs found in mobile phones and Voice over IP (VoIP) links, and even things as simple as mis-placement of the microphone). These issues can have a significant effect on the signal, especially if the person doing the recording is careless or not technically skilled.

If new methods of analysing the data are to be useful in a practical clinical environment, they need to be immune to the many types of variability encountered in the outside world, so it is also important that any database, whether for training or evaluation, is diverse enough to reflect at least some of that variability.

4.2 Effects of Coding and Transmission

The databases used during the development of new analysis systems have almost invariably been recorded either directly into digital form, or converted to digital from analogue tape recordings. In both cases, they have been stored using a lossless format to ensure that no significant features of the signal are lost.

However, especially in the case of tele-monitoring applications, there are a number of significant effects introduced by transmission, whether over analogue or lossy digital channels such as Voice over IP (VoIP) or mobile phone networks. Data can be lost due to network congestion in packet-switched networks ("packet loss"), or it can be deliberately omitted by a lossy codec to reduce the transmitted data rate.

Reilly et al. (2004) investigated the effect of long-distance analogue transmission on pathology detection. They used the MEEI database, but down-sampled it to a 10 kHz sample rate, and produced results at nearly 90 % for high quality recordings, dropping just below 75 % for the same speech transmitted over long-distance analogue telephone lines. Their results are shown in Table 4.1, together with results from (Dibazar et al. 2002), who used a very similar approach, but without down-sampling.

It is clear from these results that merely limiting the bandwidth of the speech (an unavoidable side-effect of down-sampling) approximately doubles the error rate. That rate is more than doubled again when the speech is transmitted over long-distance telephone lines, even without any simulation of background noise or handset-handling noises or distortions. It is to be expected that results from speech

Table 4.1 Comparison of results obtained on the MEEI database, processed to simulate different collection conditions

Reference (year)	Conditioning	Accuracy (%)
Reilly et al. (2004)	Telephone quality	74.2
Reilly et al. (2004)	10 kHz sampling	89.1
Dibazar et al. (2002)	Unprocessed	95.9

All results were obtained using systems based on linear discriminant classification of MDVP-like parameters

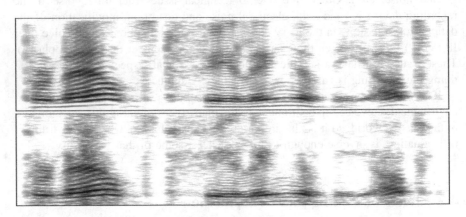

Fig. 4.1 Narrow-band spectrograms of a male speaker before GSM encoding (*upper panel*) and after (*lower panel*), showing how some frequencies are attenuated differently at different times. The sample rate was 8 kHz and the spectrograms cover the range of frequencies 0–4 kHz. The duration is 1.3 s, and the words spoken were "(a) ... pronounced feeling of the ut... (-most respect)"

collected remotely over a real telephone network would suffer a further degradation as a result of background noise, inconsistent microphone placement, handset variations, and other such factors.

For digital transmission, the corruption and distortion of the speech signal is different from the analogue case, but there is still a reduction in signal bandwidth, and there are still significant data losses. For example, lossy codecs reduce the amount of data transmitted over the mobile phone or IP network by removing redundant information and any inaudible components from the signal. They do this by using a relatively simple model of auditory perception to estimate a threshold of audibility. An example of this can be seen in Fig. 4.1.

The upper spectrogram shows the lossless signal (digitised using 16-bit linear PCM), while the lower spectrogram is the GSM-encoded version. It is apparent that some time–frequency regions have been omitted by the GSM codec. These missing components are not very audible to the human ear, but their absence will distort any MFCC or other data derived from the signal, and that distortion can be quite large. In particular, any analysis that utilises the log-power spectrum (such as cepstral analysis) can be particularly badly affected, since the very small powers in the missing frequency bands may be converted to very large negative values by the log operation. These very large values can dominate the respective signal representation, effectively destroying any useful information contained in the other frequency bands.

Remedial measures can be taken to reduce the severity of this effect, but they are rarely completely effective and generally involve a trade-off between robustness to distortion and performance on clean, undistorted speech. One example is the "floor" which is often applied to the log power spectrum during MFCC calculations. The tuning of this floor to the particular characteristics of any evaluation data can have a critical effect on the measured performance of an algorithm, but as a result, that measurement will not necessarily represent true performance in an unpredictable acoustic environment.

Since the idea was first proposed, there have been significant developments in the area of speech recognition based on representations with "missing data" (Barker et al. 2000; Cooke 2006; Joshi and Guan 2006, for example), and this approach appears to offer the greatest hope for robust analysis of this type of real-world signal. However, this is still far from being a "solved problem".

The most difficult part of the missing-data approach is normally the identification of exactly which time–frequency regions are missing or corrupted. In the case of lossy-encoded data, it is theoretically possible to estimate the "mask" from a knowledge of the codec's behaviour. In practice it is generally safe to assume that only the low-energy regions should be considered as potentially "missing".

The amount of data lost or omitted can vary between one phone call and another, or even within a call. The limited bandwidth of telephone speech (whether limited by traditional analogue electrical circuitry, or by a narrow-band digital codec) can be viewed as just another factor giving rise to such "missing data". Network congestion can result in different numbers of lost packets, and some codecs, such as the Adaptive Multi-Rate codec family (AMR-NB, AMR-WB, etc.), can change the amount of data omitted during a call, in order to match available resources.

It has long been known that missing data due to packet loss (as with mobile phones in areas of anything less than high signal strength) can have a severe effect on recognition accuracy in ASR systems (James and Milner 2006). The effects of packet loss can be ameliorated if the codec implements packet-loss concealment (PLC), but the accuracy of speech recognition still suffers if there is any significant data loss. For example (Pearce 2005) summarised the results of the Aurora project, including the effects of both codec and packet losses. He reported a relative increase in speech recognition error rate of 73 % for the AMR codec, and 159 % for EVRC, and noted that the word error rate more than doubled when the GSM signal strength fell from "strong" to "medium".

Broun et al. (2001) applied the Aurora system to *speaker* recognition rather than *speech* recognition, and found it to perform well, indicating that the front end retains at least some of the speaker-specific information which is also needed for speech pathology monitoring.

4.3 Signal Analysis

Once the speech signal has been captured, transmitted, and/or stored in digital form, many different features can be detected and quantified. Some of these are inherently low-level features, derived directly from the signal without reference to any higher-level context. To provide consistent performance, such low-level features generally need to be applied either to controlled speech (e.g. the commonly-used sustained phonation of a specific vowel), or be averaged over a relatively long period of "free" or read speech.

Other features proposed in the literature require more complicated analysis in order to extract prosodic or phonological information. Such higher-level analysis can be more sensitive to any distortion by technical factors such as the encoding/decoding process, or disruption of the speech signal by environmental factors such as background noise or distractions, so it is especially important that high-level analyses are evaluated using realistic data.

4.3.1 Pitch Estimation

Many papers, including Hariharan et al. (2010), have noted that "pitch, jitter, shimmer, the harmonics-to-noise (HNR), and the normalized noise energy" are all proven to be good indicators of vocal fold pathology, but are reliant on good pitch estimates. This is true of many other features that have been used to analyse speech pathologies as well.

Jo (2010), for example, used a small database of Korean speech (the Korean Disordered Voice Database from Changwon National University, Korea) and estimated the glottal waveform using the method from Alku (1992). His data was probably insufficient for reliable conclusions, but he found jitter and the MDVP^{TM} "Relative Average Perturbation" feature were better at identification of polyps and similar pathologies, than glottal waveform parameters. Both these parameters require accurate pitch estimation.

There is, as usual, a scarcity of standard databases for developing and evaluating pitch estimation algorithms. Plante et al. (1995) described one such database, designed specifically for evaluating pitch detectors, but it (like virtually all others) does not include pathological speech. This means that algorithms which have been developed using standard databases may not behave well when presented with speech which has unusually high levels of jitter, shimmer, breathiness or other pathology-related features.

There are further difficulties because many disorders are significantly more common in juvenile subjects, where both the pitch and the phonemic articulation are not well-matched to those used during development of the respective analysis algorithms. For example, formant frequencies are notoriously difficult to estimate from children's speech. Figure 4.2 shows the spectrum of a child's vowel with a

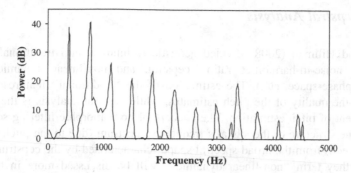

Fig. 4.2 A typical power spectrum extracted from a short segment of a child's speech with a fundamental frequency around 375 Hz. The spectral envelope defining the formant frequencies and bandwidths is ambiguous because of the spacing between pitch harmonics—it is unclear whether adjacent harmonics are the result of two closely-spaced narrow-bandwidth formants, or a single one with a large bandwidth

pitch of approximately 375 Hz. It is clear from this that there is significant ambiguity in the exact location of any formant peaks, simply because of the spacing between the pitch harmonics.

Despite this, on a cursory examination, many analyses appear to generate well-behaved pitch contours, and so appear as though they might be robust and suitable for use in analysing pathological speech. However, they often achieve this apparent level of robustness at the expense of poor responsiveness to irregularities in the glottal signal—in many cases the raw pitch estimates are deliberately filtered to suppress any rapid variations, but it is those rapid variations which are most indicative of many speech disorders. This aspect of pitch estimation (response to transient pitch irregularities) is less commonly reported than any overall bias or variation about the "true" pitch.

It has been observed that methods which produce an average estimate for jitter are statistically biased, and tend to underestimate it (Schoentgen and de Guchteneere 1995). Jitter measured using techniques such as that proposed in Vasilakis and Stylianou (2009) have been found to be better correlated with pathology than those from Praat or MDVP™.

Additionally, Titze (1994) asserts that methods using pitch of continuous speech can be unreliable for moderate to severe dysphonia, because of the large variations in pitch at voice-onset and voice-termination.

To avoid the problem of accurately identifying pitch events (i.e. glottal opening and/or closure), some research has utilised additional information, other than the acoustic signal. Some use electro-glottograph (EGG) recordings, while Gracco (1992) includes externally observable articulator movement, concentrating on the lips and jaw, using a range of different measurement systems. However, from the point of view of a telemonitoring application, it is far more convenient to use only the acoustic waveform.

4.3.2 Cepstral Analysis

Mehta and Hillman (2008) divided acoustic techniques into traditional (jitter, shimmer, noise-to-harmonics ratio), cepstral, and non-linear dynamics (e.g. entropy, phase-space, etc.). The estimation of the "traditional" features is governed by the quality of the pitch estimates, while cepstral analysis is the natural complement of pitch estimation. The concept of homomorphic filtering separates out the fine structure of the signal's frequency spectrum (due to the pitch/voicing of the speech) from the broad spectral shape (characterised by the cepstrum). The methods they term "non-linear dynamics" will be discussed more in the next section.

There are a number of potential advantages to the cepstral peak prominence (CPP) and other cepstral measures, in that they are concisely and mathematically defined, with a certain amount of robustness built-in by design.

The CPP parameter is also described in many other papers, including (Keating and Esposito 2006), and it characterises the degree of periodicity in the signal. It is essentially performing a similar function to the harmonics-to-noise ratio, but is calculated in a more robust manner, which avoids the need for explicit identification of harmonic frequencies and is less affected by any band-limiting of the signal (which may attenuate some harmonics more than others, and often removes the fundamental completely).

However, the price of this robustness is a sensitivity to certain other aspects of the signal: it does not differentiate between possible causes of aperiodicity—jitter, shimmer, breathiness, etc.—and so CPP might be expected be a robust measure of the degree of any speech disorder, but less successful at discriminating between different forms of disordered speech.

By contrast, the performance of the "traditional" techniques is more dependent on the specific details of the implementations, and especially the accuracy of the estimates of the glottal closure instants. Thus, although they have the potential to differentiate between some aspects of the signal which cannot be resolved with CPP, they tend to be more susceptible to disruption by differences in the recording environment (background noise, reverberation, encoding distortion, etc., as discussed in the following sections).

Vasilakis and Stylianou (2009) used a spectral jitter estimator to obtain short-term jitter, which they claimed to be robust against pitch errors. High jitter values became more common in pathological speech as time went on. It may be inferred from their results that the level of jitter in "normal" speech tends to remain constant.

Masaki (2010) discusses common analysis methods and the reasons why both cepstral and spectral methods are more difficult for high-pitched voices. She also describes the method that Praat uses to find pitch using the peak of the autocorrelation function, and suggests that the only real difference between cepstral peak prominence algorithm (CPP) and Murphy's "First Rahmonic Amplitude" (R1) is that R1 uses pitch-synchronous time windows.

4.3.3 Other Approaches

Many other signal processing algorithms have been applied to the detection or classification of speech disorders. There are too many to list in detail, but the few unusual methods described here may help to give an idea of the range of approaches which have been used.

Rather than analysing what is normally considered to be the speech signal itself, Castillo-Guerra and Lee (2008) describes a method for measuring timing of inspiration. They developed a text-independent algorithm with an accuracy of 84.4 %. The parameters that produced the best results were the "number of audible inspirations", the "duration of inspiration", and the average power of the "audible inspirations". Another parameter they investigated (the ratio between the maximum peak and the preceding trough of the signal power) was, however, not helpful.

Dubuisson et al. (2011) used the ratio of low-to-high frequency energy and the discontinuity at glottal closure. Using a GMM, with classification based on the majority of the analysed frames, they found about 97 % correct classification of pathological vs. normal speech taken from the MEEI database.

The non-linear dynamics methods already mentioned in respect to Mehta and Hillman (2008) have only been applied to disordered speech in relatively recent years, and are discussed in more detail in the next chapter. They have a number of characteristics which differentiate them from traditional methods, and this makes a direct comparison somewhat more difficult.

4.4 Speech and Speaker Recognition

Some approaches to the assessment of articulation in particular, have used existing automatic speech recognition (ASR) systems and quantified articulation accuracy in terms of the posterior probabilities calculated during hidden Markov model (HMM) recognition, or in terms of the estimated intelligibility of the speech, based on the recognition accuracy. Others have used alternative recognition technologies, most commonly finite state transducer (FST) and artificial neural network (ANN) systems.

Maier et al. (2009) used automatic speech recognition (ASR) and prosodic analysis, but many other approaches have been developed to make use of speech and speaker recognition methods. Speech recognition systems, sometimes configured to perform "forced alignment", "keyword spotting", or even pitch modelling, rather than full (unconstrained) speech recognition, have been used to identify the timings of specific phonemes, or to identify pitch profiles of sentences, to allow other statistics to be calculated. In some cases simple dynamic time warping (DTW, as used in very early ASR systems) is used to align two or more examples of the same spoken words.

In many cases, it is not ideal to use an 'off-the-shelf' commercial ASR system for this kind of work: for example a number of disorders are most commonly diagnosed or monitored only in very young or very old subjects, but commercial ASR systems are not optimised for performance on such voices.

Nonetheless, Shriberg et al. (2004) decided to use high-quality adult-trained HMM aligner rather than one trained specifically on children's speech because they only needed vowel/consonant discrimination and thought it better to have a more fully trained recogniser based on somewhat atypical data, rather than an inadequately trained system based on more representative data. Unfortunately, this paper's results may not be statistically significant because it appears to be a preliminary study based on only two speakers. Thus it is not clear whether their decision was justified.

4.5 Combining Statistics

It is rare for a single measure or statistic to provide sufficient discrimination to differentiate between normal and disordered speech, let alone between the different forms of disordered speech. It is therefore commonplace to calculate a large number of features, and then combine them to form a decision space with a lower dimensionality. The dimensionality of the decision space can be reduced using a linear transformation based on linear discriminant analysis (LDA), principal component analysis (PCA), or other methods such as the Sammon mapping (Sammon 1969).

However, many measures exhibit strong but non-linear correlations, and so non-linear dimensionality-reduction/classification techniques are expected to perform better. These can be based on support vector machine (SVM, essentially a form of radial basis function network, or RBFN, designed specifically for two-way pattern classification, rather than functional approximation), multi-layer perceptron (MLP), or other technologies, and have been investigated by many researchers.

There is generally some doubt about the optimality of non-linear dimensionality reduction using multi-layer neural networks because of the presence of multiple local optima. In general, it cannot be guaranteed that the training algorithm will be able to locate the global optimum, even if one exists and is unique. In this respect, SVMs and RBFNs can be optimised analytically, given sufficient training data, sufficient numerical precision and sufficient processing time. SVMs and RBFNs do however require a priori specification of specific kernel functions (Haykin 1999), and the choice of these functions, and the size of the network, cannot be guaranteed optimal (according to (Hastie et al. 2009), SVMs are known to be sensitive to choice of control parameters).

For both linear and non-linear transformations, there is a danger of over-fitting to the training data, especially if the transformation has too many degrees of freedom or the quantity or diversity of the data is insufficient. Most of the currently

Table 4.2 Summary of pathology detection results, obtained on the MEEI database, or subsets thereof

Reference (year)	Accuracy (%)
Godino-Llorente and Gómez-Vilda (2004)	95
Hadjitodorov and Mitev (2002)	96.1
Dubuisson et al. (2011)	96.7
Markaki and Stylianou (2009)	97.8
Alpan et al. (2010)	98.1
Hariharan et al. (2010)	98.5
Parsa and Jamieson (2000)	98.7
Dibazar et al. (2002)	99.4
Henríquez et al. (2009)	99.7

available disordered speech databases are still neither large nor diverse enough to support division into separate test and training sets, and still provide enough data for anything but relatively simple transformations.

4.6 Databases and Standardisation

To quote "the rule of 30" from Doddington et al. (2000), assuming each test is effectively sampled independently from a simple binomial distribution, "to be 90 % confident that a true error rate is within ±30 % of the observed error rate, there must be at least 30 errors". This suggests that even the full MEEI database contains too few speakers (700) for comparing systems with error rates below 4 %. This criterion becomes even more problematic if only a subset of the database is used, as is often done to equalise demographics between normal and pathological subjects—say 225–230 speakers, with approximately 75 % exhibiting pathologies. In this case, any observed error rates below 13 % will not be reliable (to ±30 %).

This is a severe problem for the MEEI database, because numerous papers are now reporting pathology detection rates close to, or even above, 99 % (as shown in Table 4.2). For example, Dibazar et al. (2002), who used 700 speakers from the MEEI database, achieved 99.4 % correct classification rates for discrimination of normal and pathological speech from sustained/a/phonations, while Henríquez et al. (2009) reported 99.7 % accuracy using non-linear dynamics measures (different forms of entropy and correlation dimension).

Even in the case of North American English, currently the most extensively recorded language, the quantity and diversity of data currently available is clearly insufficient to accurately test, let alone train, a functional ASR system. This precludes reliable estimation of a generic pathological speech model for most if not all speech disorders. In addition, phonetic and/or phonological labelling of what limited data is available would be needed to properly differentiate between phonetic and acoustic aspects of the different conditions. There are virtually no

databases of disordered speech outside the USA with more than some tens of
speakers. When the number of possible pathologies is taken into account, along
with the range of speaker variability (gender, age, language, accent, level of
education, etc.) it is clear that the number of speakers should exceed that used for
conventional ASR, many-fold. In practice, the opposite is the case.

Other limitations of the MEEI database, as currently supplied by
KayPENTAX® as part of the DVDP product, are partly due to the rationale behind
its design. It is not primarily intended as a database for training or assessing
automatic systems, but rather as a training aid for speech and language therapists
and other clinical practitioners. Therefore, the range of speakers has been chosen
to include a wide range of organic, neurological, traumatic, psychogenic, and other
voice disorders. This is simultaneously the database's greatest strength, and its
greatest weakness. The diversity of conditions makes the database relevant to a
wide range of different research topics, but there are a limited number of examples
corresponding to any specific diagnosis, making the training and evaluation of
specialised diagnostic aids more difficult.

The MEEI data appears to have been selected to show clear-cut examples of the
various disorders, and so, as mentioned previously, there is a scarcity of "lightly
pathological" data (Henríquez et al. 2009).

In addition, the data appears to have been selected and processed to demonstrate to a medical practitioner how to identify the different disorders. For
example, the vowel samples in the database appear to include only the stable part
of the phonation (Medida 2009) and so do not realistically represent the signals
that would be available to a telemonitoring or diagnostic aid.

There are significant differences between the way normal and disordered speech
are represented in the database. Some of these have been noted by other
researchers, but there are others as well.

Firstly, the normal speech samples are sampled at a rate of 50 kHz, but the
pathological speech samples were sampled at 25 kHz. Even if the "normal" data
were to be down-sampled to the same rate, at least some small differences will
remain between the respective signals.

Secondly, the duration of the sustained vowel phonation samples is roughly 3 s
for normal speakers, but only 1 s for pathological speakers. The disordered
speakers generally have difficulty maintaining sounds, for much longer than this,
but the systematic pre-editing of the recordings could either give any new algorithm an unrealistic advantage, or it could conceal features which might otherwise
be exploited to improve performance.

Finally, the Rainbow Passage recordings were limited to 12 s in duration,
regardless of the speaking rate of the individual speaker. Since dysarthric speakers
often have significantly lower speaking rates than normal speakers, there will be a
systematic difference between the phonetic content of the disordered speech
recordings and the normal ones, and a new algorithm might well respond to those
differences, giving it an unrealistic advantage.

To quote (Malyska et al. 2005), "a problem with MEEI database is that some of
the normal speakers were recorded at different sites and over potentially different

channels than the pathological voices. This could explain the better performance of voice pathology detection system(s) on (the) MEEI (data)—as well as the larger degradation when the same system is tested on a different database."

Vasilakis and Stylianou (2009) compared Praat, MDVP^{TM} and their own "SJE" method for estimating jitter, with a view to analysing running speech rather than sustained vowels. They evaluated on the MEEI database and another, the "Príncipe de Asturias (PdA) Hospital in Alcalá de Henares of Madrid" database. Like (Henríquez et al. 2009), they found much better performance on MEEI than their own database, possibly for the same reason hypothesised in Henríquez et al. (2009)—that the MEEI database contains no "lightly pathological" speakers, and thus does not present a realistic level of difficulty in this task.

In the second "multi-quality" database used by Henríquez et al., the speakers fell into four groups: healthy, and light, moderate, or severe pathology, not just two, healthy and pathological, as in the MEEI data.

Vasilakis and Stylianou reported accuracies between 90 and 95 % on the MEEI data, but only between 63 and 85 % on the PdA database (depending on the parameters being used). This difference between evaluation on the MEEI data, and that on other databases used for cross-validation, is very typical of the published literature. Most reported pathology detection accuracies for MEEI data are in excess of 95 %, but those on other databases rarely exceed 85 %.

Ferguson et al. (2009) discusses the shortcomings of databases tailored to a particular task, in a linguistic rather than acoustic context, while Hariharan et al. (2010) also mentions the difficulty of comparison with other published results due to differences in methodology and data.

A summary of some results obtained on both the MEEI and other databases are summarised in Table 4.3. In general, excluding the Silva (dympJitt/dympLocJitt) result, the MEEI data gives accuracy figures about 13 % higher than the other databases. However, the results from (Silva et al. 2009) suggest an alternative explanation for this apparent bias. They found that the optimum analysis method was different for the MEEI data, from that for the DB02. Using their best method for the MEEI data gave a bias of 18 % absolute toward the MEEI result. Using the best method for the DB02 database, gave a bias of 17 % toward *that* database. Thus, it appears that, for Silva et al.'s methods at least, the bias in favour of results from the MEEI database might be due simply to the optimisation of the methods for performance on that data. If the methods had been chosen or designed to optimise performance on other data, the observed bias might well be reversed.

Despite these issues, the MEEI database has proven to be of great value in this field, and is still the largest and most diverse database that is readily available. It is likely to remain the de-facto standard database for evaluation and comparison of disordered speech analysis systems for the foreseeable future. Nonetheless, it is still critically important to evaluate any algorithms on data recorded independently from that used during the design/training phase (Sáenz-Lechón et al. 2006).

Tsanas et al. (2012) makes references to possible over-fitting of the system to the training data, but despite this, their results seem quite respectable. It does

Table 4.3 Comparison of results obtained on the MEEI database with other databases

Reference (year)	Method	MEEI accuracy (%)	Other accuracy (%) (database)
Silva et al. (2009)	dympJitt dympLocJitt	71	88 (DB02)
Silva et al. (2009)	dympSTJEa	87	69 (DB02)
Vasilakis and Stylianou (2009)		94.8	84.7 (PdA)
Markaki and Stylianou (2009)		97.8	90.2 (PdA)
Henríquez et al. (2009)		99.7	82.5 (Multiquality)

The DB02 database is described in Silva et al. (2009), the Príncipe de Asturias Hospital in Alcalá de Henares of Madrid (PdA) database in Godino-Llorente et al. (2008), and the "Multiquality" database in Alonso et al. (2001). The accuracy on the MEEI data is an average of 7.18 % higher than the others

demonstrate though, that a greater quantity and variety of data would make the efficacy of different techniques more unequivocal.

In Sáenz-Lechón et al. (2006), there is an informative summary of others work. For their own work, they use a similar subset of the MEEI database to that in Parsa and Jamieson (2000), which is balanced for distributions of gender and age between 173 pathological and 53 normal speakers.

They use both detector error trade-off (DET) curves (as used in speaker verification and identification, SVI) and receiver operating characteristic (ROC) curves (as in medical decision-making systems), pointing out that the DET makes comparison between the "folds" of a K-fold cross-validation clearer and that the "curves" are more close to straight lines in the DET, making them easier to compare with a simple linear discrimination.

Pützer and Koreman (1997) describes a German database. Out of 95 speakers, two had symptoms from more than one category. They collected a read text and the vowels /i/, /a/ and /u/, and included electro-glottograph (EGG) waveforms. They also recorded the phoniatric diagnoses based on video recordings of the vocal folds.

The paper (Castillo-Guerra and Lee 2008), which used timing of inspiration, supplemented the MEEI database with two others from Darley et al. (1975) and Castillo-Guerra and Méndez Rodríguez (2001).

References

Alku P (1992) Glottal wave analysis with pitch synchronous Interactive adaptive inverse filtering. Speech Commun 11:109–118

Alonso JB, de León J, Alonso I, Ferrer MA (2001) Automatic detection of pathologies in the voice by HOS based parameters. EURASIP J Appl Signal Process 2001:275–284

Alpan A, Schoentgen J, Maryn Y, Grenez F (2010) Automatic perceptual categorization of disordered connected speech. In: Proceedings of 11th annual conference on international speech communication association 2010, pp 2574–2577

Bakker K, Arkebauer H, Boutsen F (1993) Computer-assisted determination of diadochokinetic rate and variability. Mini-seminar presented at annual convention of the American Speech and Hearing Association (ASHA). http://www.sph.sc.edu/Documents/1997ASHAhandout.pdf. Accessed 16 Feb 2012

Barker J, Josifovski L, Cooke M, Green P (2000) Soft decisions in missing data techniques for robust automatic speech recognition. In Proceedings of the international conference on speech and language processing ICSLP-2000, pp 373–376

Boersma P, Weenink D (2009) Praat: doing phonetics by computer. http://www.praat.org/. Accessed 16 Feb 2012

Broun CC, Campbell WM, Pearce D, Kelleher H (2001) Distributed speaker recognition using the ETSI distributed speech recognition standard. In: Proceedings of international conference on artificial intelligence ICAI-2001, vol 1, pp 244–248

Castillo-Guerra E, Lee W (2008) Automatic acoustics measurement of audible inspirations in pathological voices.: In Proceedings of acoustics-08, pp 3661–3666

Castillo-Guerra E, Méndez Rodríguez NL (2001) Methodology for obtaining a pathological dysarthric speech database. In Proceedings of 7th international symposium on social communication

Cooke M (2006) A glimpsing model of speech perception in noise. J Acoust Soc Amer 119(3):1562–1573

Darley FL, Aronson AE, Brown JR (1975) Motor speech disorders. W. B. Saunders, Philadelphia

Dibazar AA, Narayanan S, Berger TW (2002) Feature analysis for automatic detection of pathological speech. Eng Med and Biol 2002: In: 24th annual conference and the annual fall meeting of the biomedical engineering society embs/bmes conference, vol 1, pp 182–183. doi:10.1109/IEMBS.2002.1134447

Doddington GR, Przybocki MA, Martin AF, Reynolds DA (2000) The NIST speaker recognition evaluation—overview, methodology, systems, results, perspective. Speech Commun 31(2–3):225–254

Dubuisson T, Drugman T, Dutoit T (2011) On the use of grey zones in automatic voice pathology detection. In Proceedings of 9th Pan-Eur Voice Conference (PEVOC9). http://tcts.fpms.ac.be/~drugman/files/pevoc9-VoicePatho.pdf. Accessed 16 Feb 2012

Ferguson A, Craig H, Spencer E (2009) Exploring the potential for corpus-based research in speech-language pathology. In Selected proceedings of the 2008 HCSNet workshop on designing the Australian National Corpus: Mustering Languages:30–36

Godino-Llorente JI, Gómez-Vilda P (2004) Automatic detection of voice impairments by means of short-term cepstral parameters and neural network based detectors. IEEE Trans Biomed Eng 51(2):380–384

Godino-Llorente JI, Osma-Ruiz V, Sáenz-Lechón N, Cobeta-Marco I, González-Herranz R, Ramírez-Calvo C (2008) Acoustic analysis of voice using WPCVox: a comparative study with multi dimensional voice program. Eur Arch Otolaryngol 265:465–476

Gracco VL (1992) Analysis of speech movements: practical considerations and clinical application. Haskins Laboratories status report on speech research SR-109/110, pp 45–58

Hadjitodorov S, Mitev P (2002) A computer system for acoustic analysis of pathological voices and laryngeal diseases screening. Med Eng Phys 24:419–429

Hariharan M, Paulraj MP, Yaacob S (2010) Time-domain features and probabilistic neural network for the detection of vocal fold pathology. Malays J Comput Sci 23(1):60–67

Hastie T, Tibshirani R, Friedman J (2009) The elements of statistical learning: data mining, inference, and prediction, 2nd edn. Springer, Heidelberg

Haykin S (1999) Neural networks: a comprehensive foundation. Prentice Hall International, New Jersey

Henríquez P, Alonso JB, Ferrer MA, Travieso CM, Godino-Llorente JI, Díaz-de-María F (2009) Characterization of healthy and pathological voice through measures based on nonlinear dynamics. IEEE Trans Audio Speech Lang Process 17(6):1186–1195

James A, Milner B (2006) Towards improving the robustness of distributed speech recognition in packet loss. Speech Commun 48:1402–1421. doi:10.1016/j.specom.2006.07.005

Jo C (2010) Source analysis of pathological voice. In: Proceedings of the international multiconference of engineers and computer scientists, vol 2, 1271–1274

Joshi N, Guan L (2006) Missing data ASR with fusion of features and combination of recognizers. In Proceedings of IEEE spoken language technology workshop 2006, pp 114–117. doi:10.1109/SLT.2006.326830

Keating PA, Esposito C (2006) Linguistic voice quality. UCLA Working Pap Phon 105:85–91

Maier A, Haderlein T, Eysholdt U, Rosanowski F, Batliner A, Schuster M, Nöth E (2009) PEAKS—a system for the automatic evaluation of voice and speech disorders. Speech Commun 51(5):425–437. doi:10.1016/j.specom.2009.01.004

Malyska N, Quatieri TF, Sturim D (2005) Automatic dysphonia recognition using biologically inspired amplitude-modulation features. In: IEEE international conference on acoustics, speech and signal processing ICASSP-2005, pp 873–876

Markaki M, Stylianou Y (2009) Using modulation spectra for voice pathology detection and classification. In Proceedings of IEEE Conference on Engineering in Medicine and Biology Society 2009, pp 2514–2517

Masaki A (2010) Optimizing acoustic and perceptual assessment of voice quality in children with vocal nodules. PhD thesis, Harvard-MIT Health Sciences and Technology

Medida P (2009) Spectral analysis of pathological acoustic speech waveforms. MSc Thesis, University of Nevada, Las Vegas

Mehta DD, Hillman RE (2008) Voice assessment: updates on perceptual, acoustic, aerodynamic, and endoscopic imaging methods. Curr Opin in Otolaryngol Head Neck Surg 16(3):211–215. doi:10.1097/MOO.0b013e3282fe96ce

Parsa V, Jamieson DG (2000) Identification of pathological voices using glottal noise measures. J Speech Lang Hearing Res 43(2):469–485

Pearce D (2005) Distributed speech recognition. http://www.w3.org/2005/05/DSR.pdf. Accessed 16 Feb 2012

Plante F, Meyer GF, Ainsworth WA (1995) A pitch extraction reference database. In: Proceeding of 4th european conference on speech communication and technology-1995, pp 837–840

Pützer M, Koreman J (1997) A German database of patterns of pathological vocal fold vibration. PHONUS 3:143–153

Reilly RB, Moran R, Lacy PD (2004) Voice pathology assessment based on a dialogue system and speech analysis. In: Proceedings of American association for artificial intelligence fall symposium on dialog systems for health communication, pp 104–109

Sáenz-Lechón N, Godino-Llorente JI, Osma-Ruiz V, Gómez-Vilda P (2006) Methodological issues in the development of automatic systems for voice pathology detection. Biomed Signal Process Control 1(2):120–128

Sammon JW (1969) A nonlinear mapping for data structure analysis. IEEE Trans Comput 18:401–409

Schoentgen J, de Guchteneere R (1995) Time series analysis of jitter. J Phon 23:189–201

Shriberg LD, Hosom J-P, Green JR (2004) Diagnostic assessment of childhood apraxia of speech using automatic speech recognition (ASR) systems. J Med Speech Lang Pathol 12(4):167–171

Silva DG, Oliveira LC, Andrea M (2009) Jitter estimation algorithms for detection of pathological voices. EURASIP J Adv Signal Process 2009:1–10. doi:10.1155/2009/567875

Sjölander K (2004) The snack sound toolkit http://www.speech.kth.se/snack/. Accessed 16 Feb 2012

Sutton S, Cole RA, de Villiers J, Schalkwyk J, Vermeulen PJE, Macon MW, Yan Y, Kaiser EC, Rundle B, Shobaki K, Hosom J-P, Kain A, Wouters J, Massaro DW, Cohen MM (1998) Universal speech tools: the CSLU toolkit. In: Proceedings of international conference on spoken language processing ICSLP-98:3221–3224

Titze IR (1994) Summary statement. National center for voice and speech workshop on acoustic voice analysis. http://www.ncvs.org/freebooks/summary-statement.pdf. Accessed 16 Feb 2012

Tsanas A, Little MA, McSharry PE, Spielman J, Ramig LO (2012) Novel speech signal processing algorithms for high-accuracy classification of Parkinson's disease. IEEE Trans Biomed Eng 59(5):1264–1271

Vasilakis M, Stylianou Y (2009) Voice pathology detection based on short-term jitter estimations in running speech. Folia Phoniatr Logop 61(3):153–170. doi:10.1159/000219951

Chapter 5
Established Methods

Abstract Both pre-processing (feature extraction) and pattern classification techniques are discussed in this chapter. Traditionally, specialised parameters have been used for the analysis of speech disorders: harmonic-to-noise ratio, jitter, shimmer, and others. These have been devised using expert opinions from speech and language therapists and other professionals. They are typically calculated using widely available software packages, but still require trained personnel to collect and prepare the recordings, as well as to interpret the resulting parameters. More recently, researchers have also investigated many of the parameters or features used in speech and speaker recognition. Features such as the ubiquitous mel-frequency cepstral coefficients are often used, but so are numerous less common methods, such as formant frequencies, modulation spectra, chaos-theory parameters, and prosodic and phonological features. Each of these has had its fair share of success, but the most successful systems have generally used a combination of multiple features and/or multiple classification algorithms. Numerous methods for discriminating between disordered and normal speech, and sometimes between different forms of speech disorder, have been devised. They have typically been based on neural networks, Markov models, support vector machines, and other classifiers (both linear and non-linear), although Gaussian Mixture Models are probably the most widely used, robust, and successful so far.

Keywords Complementary features · Discrimination and transformation · Pitch estimation accuracy · Statistically optimised classification

Most methods for classifying disordered speech rely on the characteristics of individual speech sounds to make their decision. Thus they either operate on sustained phonations, where the whole utterance can be analysed as a single unit, or divide the signal into a sequence of very short segments before calculating parameters describing each segment individually. Both these approaches yield

L. Baghai-Ravary and S. W. Beet, *Automatic Speech Signal Analysis for Clinical Diagnosis and Assessment of Speech Disorders*, SpringerBriefs in Speech Technology, DOI: 10.1007/978-1-4614-4574-6_5, © The Author(s) 2013

what can be considered as "local features", describing characteristics of the specific sounds being produced at a specific point in time.

Discriminating between some conditions, however, is potentially easier if extended recordings of natural speech communication can be analysed. In this case, a third approach is also possible, where "global features" are calculated, describing overall characteristics of the speech, rather than those specific to a particular point in time. Possible global features include the rapidity and precision of transitions from one speech sound to the next, and the ranges of the formant frequencies, the pitch, and/or the speaking rate.

5.1 Features

Virtually all attempts to analyse characteristics of speech or to classify it in any way, start by forming an intermediate representation of the original waveform. The aim of this pre-processing is to enhance the features of interest, and suppress other forms of variability, whether due to background noise, distortion, reverberation, or the inherent variability of human speech production. Some of the more well-established and popular representations or 'local features' are discussed below.

5.1.1 Cepstral Analysis

Dibazar et al. (2002) used MFCCs and pitch in an HMM. They experimented with the Rainbow Passage, but discrimination was slightly worse than with the sustained /a/ data. They also tried MDVP^{TM} parameters supplied with the MEEI database and different classifiers (of which, GMM was the best), but again they were slightly worse than the MFCC and pitch parameters, which are also easier to calculate. They didn't attempt to discriminate between pathologies.

Alpan et al. (2009) described the first rahmonic (R1) amplitude measure, investigated the effects of window length and other parameters, and compared it with CPP. They found a 73 % correlation between R1 amplitude and human ratings (on the 4-point GRABS scale), by applying a 2 kHz low-pass filter and amplitude normalisation (i.e. DC removal from the log power spectrum). Their analysis used a fixed 46 ms (2048 samples) window length.

The corresponding results for CPP gave a similar 71 % correlation. These figures might have been more informative if they had calculated the Spearman rank correlation coefficient, rather than simple linear correlation, because the "best fit" straight line to their data clearly did not pass through the origin of the graph, and there is no obvious reason to assume that any correlation with human ratings would be linear in any case. The Spearman rank correlation makes no such assumption.

Table 5.1 Summary of equal-error rates for dysphonia detection

System	Equal-error rate (%)
MFCC	3.8
ICC	5.7
MFCC + ICC fusion	2.0

As reported in Malyska et al. (2005), for MFCCs, their own "biologically-inspired modulation feature extraction system" (referred to as ICC), and a fusion of the two systems

Nonetheless, they observed that pitch synchronous analysis generally performed slightly better than fixed-window analysis, but the best overall was the fixed-window, 2 kHz low-pass filtered result.

5.1.2 Formant Tracks

Salhi et al. (2010) used multi-layer neural networks to differentiate between normal, neural and vocal pathologies (Parkinson, Alzheimer, laryngeal, dyslexia etc.). They used an in-house database, LPC-derived formant frequencies and pitch, while (Muhammad et al. 2011) analysed Arabic spoken digits from 62 dysphonic patients with six different types of voice disorders and 50 normal subjects. The distribution of the first four formants of the vowel /a/ was extracted to examine deviation of the formants from normal.

It would be expected that dysphonia would be clearly identifiable from formant frequencies, but this group found there was "large variation" within and between groups. They then attempted to use recognition accuracy as a diagnostic. The accuracy for dysphonic speech was indeed lower than that for normal speech, but did not improve following therapy, suggesting that the accuracy did not mirror the severity of the symptoms as perceived by acoustic analysis.

5.1.3 Modulation Spectra

Malyska et al. (2005) investigated modulation-based features, in the form of a mathematically defined process which had been inspired by the peripheral auditory system's sensitivity to modulation in different frequency bands. The analysis was neither an accurate, nor a complete, replication of auditory perception, having been developed from a mathematical and computational viewpoint, but did have robust numerical properties, making it well suited to automatic analysis. They obtained their best performance by fusing the results of a traditional MFCC-based system with those from their auditory-inspired modulation analysis. They used a GMM-based classification system, and concluded that the additional modulation-based data was complementary to MFCCs. Their results are summarised in Table 5.1.

Markaki and Stylianou (2009) initially took a different approach. They used radial basis functions (RBFs), singular value decomposition (SVD) and SVMs to differentiate various vocal pathologies (polyp vs. keratosis, leukoplakia, adductor spasmodic dysphonia and vocal nodules). Again, they mention the difficulty of accurate pitch estimation with some pathologies, and to avoid this problem, they started by considering the flatness of the LP-spectrum and the LP-residual. However, they did mention that other researchers have found LP parameters to be inadequate for differentiation between pathologies, and that better results had been obtained with jitter.

In an attempt to avoid this inadequacy, they went on to investigate modulation spectra (probability distributions over signal frequency and modulation frequency) and Maximal Relevance. Again they used the /a/ phonemes (the modulation spectrograms were calculated from the whole of each phoneme as represented in the MEEI database). They achieved 90 % discrimination between pathologies.

More recently Markaki et al. (2010) also concluded that their implementation of the modulation spectrum yielded information which was complementary to MFCCs, although they believed that normalisation was important. They did not compare their normalised modulation spectrum results with *normalised* MFCCs or delta MFCCs, so it cannot be stated categorically whether the complementarity of their data was due to its characterisation of modulation, due to the normalisation process, or due to the representation capturing dynamic aspects of the signal.

This is one of relatively few papers which trained the recogniser on one database (PdA) and tested on another completely separate one (MEEI). It might have been enlightening if they had repeated the experiment with the databases reversed, so that fine levels of discrimination could be tested. Nonetheless, the use of full cross-database validation is to be commended.

5.1.4 Prosodic Features

Llerena et al. (2011) states "Pitch detection is one of the most difficult problems encountered when analysing speech signals" but it does not appear to suggest that pathological speech is more difficult that normal, apart from the statement that "(pathological) speech signals are degraded because of unavoidable external factors like, for example, more noisy components, attenuation, disappearance of components, shifted harmonics and so on". In this paper, the authors adapted normal speech pitch estimators to pathological speech. They compared autocorrelation, harmonic product spectrum and wavelet methods. Assessment of roughness, hoarseness and breathiness was best with wavelets.

Silva et al. (2009) found, contrary to common practice, that absolute jitter (in units of time) out-performed relative jitter (expressed as a proportion of the pitch period) in the detection of physical vocal fold pathologies. They presented results for 7 different jitter evaluation methods, in both absolute and relative forms (making a total of 14 different measures) and for both the MEEI database and their own smaller database, recorded in a similar fashion. The only significant difference between the two databases is that the disordered speech in the MEEI data was recorded differently from the normal speech, as noted previously, whereas all the data in the in-house database was sampled at a single rate, 50 kHz, and with the same procedures (as far as possible). The details of the room acoustics, etc., will also have differed between the two databases, but these differences cannot be readily quantified. It is noteworthy that the relative performances of the different measures were quite different between the two databases. This may have been simple random variation due to the small size of the in-house database, or it may be because the differences mentioned above.

Awan and Scarpino (2004) compared three widely-used pitch detection algorithms (Dr Speech, Kay CSL^{TM} model 4300, and CSpeechSP) and found that although mean pitch values were very similar, the variations from the mean were very different. They quote many sources which advise against taking any automatic method at face value unless it has been validated manually. They say that this is especially relevant for male, low-pitched speech, despite the accepted wisdom that female and child speech is more difficult. They describe all this from the viewpoint of a clinician investigating pathological speech, rather than a developer of new algorithms.

Many authors (Askenfelt and Hammarberg 1986; de Krom 1995; Parsa and Jamieson 2001) assert that continuous speech is more relevant to human perception but it is not clear that that relevance will apply to automatic diagnosis and monitoring methods, where the "higher levels" of processing still fall far short of human perception and interpretation.

In practice, many measures of phonation (jitter, shimmer, harmonic-to-noise ratio etc.) are only reliable and unambiguous when applied to signals of expected frequency and intensity stability, e.g. sustained vowels (Horii 1979; Baken 1987; de Krom 1994). In most reported systems, this latter factor appears to be more important than the performance increment which human listeners can derive from continuous speech, but which still eludes automatic systems.

Ringeval (2010) used six features (low-level descriptors: ESPS pitch, energy, deltas and delta-deltas) in a Gaussian mixture model, and fused the results with recognition results based on statistical features derived from the same low level descriptors.

5.1.5 Phonological Features

Middag et al. (2009) proposed a method which they evaluated by comparing automatic with expert clinicians' estimates of intelligibility. For general speech disorders, their system resulted in a Pearson correlation of 0.86, while for dysarthria-specific system the figure was 0.94.

5.2 Temporal Models

Some methods for analysing disordered speech simply examine long-term statistics of local features, while others consider characteristics of specific parts of the speech signal (phonological classes, phonemes, syllables, or even whole sentences). Many of the latter methods therefore require some form of modelling of the temporal structure of the speech, either to identify when the respective segments of the speech start and finish, or to identify how well the disordered speech matches various models of the respective phones.

5.2.1 Hidden Markov Models

By far the most widely used acoustic-temporal model of speech is the hidden Markov model (HMM). There are many variants of HMM, and although one form is often claimed to be better or more robust than another, the superiority of any specific form is generally dependent on the details of the task at hand. In particular, the choice of HMM (or other temporal model) is dependent on:

- the quantity and diversity of data used to train the models
- the perplexity of the recognition or alignment task
- the dimensionality and other numerical characteristics of the local features (speech representation)
- the availability of computational resources, both during training and application of the methods.

Middag et al. (2009) used Spraak with MFCCs transformed into probabilities of 24 discrete phonological features, as input. Although not stated explicitly, this appears to be essentially a form of semi-continuous HMM (SC-HMM). The phonological probabilities are derived using 4 ANNs, trained on non-pathological speech. The models only had one state per phone, and were context-independent (monophone) models. The phonological features, however, were context-dependent. They used 5-fold cross-validation to decide on the best models, and RMS errors rather than Pearson correlation because the RMS error was found to be more stable across groups.

More significantly, "... the new system with only one ASR comprising 55 context-independent acoustic states achieves the same performance as our formerly published system with two ASRs, one of which is a rather complex one comprising about a thousand triphone acoustic states...". It appears that the context-dependency of the phonological features might be the key factor allowing this simultaneous reduction in complexity and increase in performance.

5.3 Classification and Discrimination

Depending on the details of the rest of the process, it is often necessary, at some stage, to either decide to which of two or more classes the speech belongs, or to calculate a simple measure of how similar one sample of speech is to another. Both of these processes can be considered as a transformation of the parameters chosen to characterise the signal, yielding a result which may be either discrete or continuous. This result may be a single value, or it may be multidimensional. The transformation of the data being discriminated between may be linear, or it can be a complicated non-linear process.

The most common methods used in publications to date include linear discriminant analysis (LDA, which is closely related to a number of other transformations such as principal component analysis, PCA), various forms of artificial neural network (ANN), and support vector machines (SVMs). There are exceptions to this generalisation, such as (Droppo and Acero 2010) which used phoneme edit-distance measures to choose a better result from a set of top-N results, taking into account the probabilities of different mispronunciations.

In general, the most successful classifiers are capable of being optimised statistically, being trained by exposure to large quantities of realistic data, and adjusting the numerous parameters which define the classification process. Carmichael et al. (2008) presented work which might, at first sight, appear to go against this general trend. They attempted the diagnosis of different forms of dysarthria using automatic methods of decision-making, based on the gradings from clinicians' Frenchay Dysarthria Assessments.

They took as a baseline, a previous (statistically optimised) approach based on linear discriminant analysis (LDA), but obtained significantly better performance using a hybrid system comprising a statistically-optimised component (a multilayer perceptron, or MLP) and a rule-based (RBC) component which was *not* statistically optimised. This hybrid approach gave approximately 40 % fewer errors than their baseline. It must be mentioned that this comparison was skewed because the RBC system had access to supplementary information which was not available to the baseline, but the improvement is also attributable to the design of the hybrid system—with the statistically optimised component able to learn, and partially correct for, any sub-optimality in the RBC component.

There have been many attempts to break away from continuous-distribution mixtures-of-Gaussians HMM (CD-HMM) recognition in recent years, including a deep neural network/HMM hybrid (DNN-HMM) (Dahl et al. 2012), semicontinuous HMMs (SC-HMMs) (Haderlein et al. 2006), and weighted finite-state transducers (WFSTs) (Pompili et al. 2011), many of which offer hope for better generalisation and more compact models.

Many papers, including Hariharan et al. (2010) have discussed the commonly-used speech analysis and classification tools, including multi-layer perceptron (MLP—probably the most widely used form of ANN), learning vector quantisation (LVQ), hidden Markov model (HMM), linear discriminant analysis (LDA),

Gaussian mixture model (GMM) and K-nearest neighbour (KNN) classifiers. The general superiority of any specific technique is, however, rarely clear-cut. One approach may appear to have clear benefits in one situation or one application, but may be inferior in another.

For example, the very thorough and detailed study reported in (Tsanas et al. 2012) looked at sustained vowels using a dysphonia measure subset taken from 132 originally computed dysphonia measures, and achieved 99 % discrimination between Parkinson's Disease and normal speech. The measures included many variants of jitter, shimmer and signal-to-noise ratio related measures. They compared four different feature selection algorithms to identify robust, parsimonious dysphonia measure subsets, and evaluated the out-of-sample performance of those subsets using Random Forests (RFs) and Support Vector Machines (SVMs) for classification. They used the National Center for Voice and Speech (NCVS) database comprising 263 phonations from 43 subjects. As usual, there was a roughly 3:1 ratio between the numbers of pathological and normal speakers. They used 10-fold cross validation, with 100 different random permutations of the original dataset to split the data into test and training sets, but all data was taken from the same database with the same recording procedures etc.

They found the RF approach was not as good as the SVM in this application, for the current dataset, and gender-specific classification wasn't as accurate as pooling together the entire dataset (i.e. without data partitioning according to gender). This slightly surprising finding is highlighted in the paper and is left as an issue worthy of further investigation using a larger database.

In the field of automatic speech recognition, this latter finding would normally be indicative of a lack of data in one or both of the gender-specific pools used for training. In that case, although an SVM system appears better than RF, when trained on gender-independent data, the same may not be true for gender or age-specific systems trained on a larger dataset.

Thus, despite the great care taken by the authors of that paper, and the impressive performance of their best system on the task they were addressing, additional tests on a larger and more varied database would be required to verify those conclusions. The availability of such additional data might also allow the gender-specific vs. gender-independent issue to be resolved more conclusively.

5.3.1 Linear Transformations and Discriminant Analysis

Castillo-Guerra and Lovey (2003) compared two methods of dysarthria assessment using features extracted from pathological speech signals. One was based on linear discriminant analysis (LDA), while the other was non-linear, based on self-organizing maps. The non-linear method was not only found to give the better classification accuracy, but it also used a 2-dimensional representation which appeared to yield additional information related to the location of any damage in the peripheral or central nervous system.

Numerous other researchers have used linear discriminant analysis to differentiate between speaker types (Reilly et al. 2004; Dibazar et al. 2002) and because of the numerical robustness of this approach, many have produced very competitive results.

5.3.2 Artificial Neural Networks

Hosom et al. (2004) compared standard methods—Lexical Stress Ratio (LSR) and the Coefficient of Variation Ratio (CVR) computed via the Kay CSL^{TM} system —with values computed via ASR to identify silence, speech, stressed and unstressed vowels, etc. Their CVR ASR was trained on a composite database collected from children with suspected apraxia of speech (AOS) over a period of 20 years. The collection of this database is in itself a major achievement. The LSR ASR was trained on adult non-pathological data, with an HMM/ANN hybrid system. They found a close agreement between automatic CVR and the system based on CSL^{TM} (within 2.7 %) and almost as good for LSR (within 6.7 %). CVR is based on conversational speech.

Salhi et al. (2010) described a small study based on a wavelet representation which was then fed into a neural network for classification, while Hariharan et al. (2010) combined the neural network paradigm with the more mathematically grounded probabilistic approach normally associated with Hidden Markov Models, focussing on the identification of vocal fold pathology. The use of specially designed local features allowed them to avoid explicit pitch detection, while the probabilistic neural networks produce results which can be utilised directly in a mathematical framework.

5.3.3 Support Vector Machines

The SVM formulation embodies the Structural Risk Minimisation (SRM) principle, as opposed to the Empirical Risk Minimisation (ERM) approach commonly employed within statistical learning methods. SRM minimises an upper bound on the generalisation error, as opposed to ERM that minimises the error on the training data. It is often stated that it is this difference that equips SVMs with a greater potential to generalise, the ultimate goal of statistical learning (Gunn 1998).

Unfortunately, this potential advantage is often dwarfed by the complexity of the system required when the input dimensionality is large, as well as the need for high-precision and time-consuming computations when calculating the system parameters.

The most practically important advantage offered by SVMs is that they can be optimised globally, and in a single pass, without the need for an iterative gradient-descent algorithm such as those used to train multi-layer neural networks, for example. Most alternative technologies are trained to minimise some form of cost function, and that cost function may contain local minima which an iterative training procedure cannot discriminate from the global minimum. As a result, these systems are rarely fully optimised, even after extensive training.

Ganapathiraju et al. (2004) describes the advantages of SVM over other competing technologies, and develops a hybrid SVM/HMM approach to speech recognition, while (Padrell-Sendra et al. 2006) uses SVMs outside the usual HMM framework.

5.4 Phase-Space Representation

The concepts of chaos and entropy were first applied to speech signals around the time of (Kumar and Mullick 1990). Soon afterwards, principles of phase-space analysis were applied to disordered speech in Accardo et al. (1992). They tackled a difficult problem: distinguishing between normal speech, ataxic dysarthria, and hyperkinetic extrapyramidal dysarthria. This multi-way classification does not usually yield nearly such high accuracies as the simple two-way decision involved in discrimination between normal and disordered speech. Since then, developments have continued, including the demonstration of the ability to (at least partially) separate noise and speech into distinct sub-spaces (Moakes and Beet 1994).

More recently, Henríquez et al. (2009) used a phase-space representation of speech with entropy measures and an ANN to discriminate between normal and pathological speech from the MEEI database. They achieved success rates of 82.5 % on an in-house multi-quality database of sustained vowels, and 99.7 % with a subset of the commercial MEEI database of sustained /a/ phonemes. This subset was chosen to have diagnosis, gender and age distributions matched between normal and pathological speakers. For the MEEI data, the vowel durations were 3 s for healthy voices and 1 s for pathological voices. Their results might show how performance can be degraded when the recording procedures and equipment change, or, as mentioned previously, it might be, as the authors suggest, that there is a lack of "lightly pathological" data in the MEEI database. They found that performance is similar on both databases if moderate and lightly pathological data is excluded. In their in-house database, they recorded five different steady vowels, but found that /a/ gave significantly better results than the others.

Also they indicate that the most important measures and algorithms in the contemporary literature use either fundamental frequency, or dynamic time warping combined with an Itakura–Saito distortion measure. The algorithms they considered give reported accuracies between 76.7 and 96.1 %. Their phase-space feature, with its 99.7 % accuracy, appears to be the best reported result to date, on the age and gender-balanced MEEI database subset at least.

However, when the measured accuracy approaches so close to 100 %, it would be highly desirable to evaluate on a much larger database: the "Rule of 30" mentioned previously suggests that the database should be large enough to produce around 30 errors, if the performance estimate is to be reliable. In the MEEI subset results quoted in Henríquez et al. (2009), there appear to have been roughly half that number, meaning that the difference in accuracy between their system and the next best, may be much less clear-cut than their results suggest.

5.5 Complete Systems

With so many alternative technologies on which to build a new system, it is hardly surprising that there have been a vast number of different systems proposed, and many have provided insights into the issues discussed in this book.

For example, Maier et al. (2010) compared ASR recognition with "expert" intelligibility ratings of head/neck cancer patients with dysglossia and/or dysphonia (average age over 60). They found that the optimum language model (in terms of the number of words, N, in the N-grams) was different for recognition accuracy than for correlation with expert assessments of intelligibility.

However, that does not imply that either the automatic approach, or the expert assessment scale, is inferior in any way—merely that better performance can be achieved by a holistic approach, and that it is unwise simply to mimic expert assessments of speech features, unless the way the experts interpret their own assessments can also be replicated.

The unusual approach described in Haderlein et al. (2006) exploited the mismatch between a standard ASR system's models, and ones optimised for the individual subject, in order to differentiate between four different speech characteristics. They mention that normal acoustic evaluation of voice disorders is done mostly using sustained phonation of specific vowel-sounds, but felt that it would be beneficial to analyse a read passage instead. They fed this into a semi-continuous HMM (SC-HMM) system, with speaker-specific models adapted from speaker-independent ones by interpolation of weights, as in Steidl et al. (2004). The "standard" speaker-independent system was trained with 27 h of speech, but the speaker-specific models used much less: between 35 s and 3 min.

They observed that this approach is computationally expensive, but found that comparisons based on standard MFCCs were not suitable for this task. They devised a distance measure between models and used a Sammon mapping (Sammon 1969) to reduce the dimensionality of the feature space. Two dimensions were found to be sufficient to separate four classes of speaker (young, old, laryngectomised, and hoarse), albeit not with simple linear boundaries between classes. Thus there was still a need for manual interpretation of the results.

Remote assessment and treatment via a broadband internet connection has been detailed in Pompili et al. (2011) which used a hybrid MLP/HMM large-vocabulary recognition engine (AUDIMUS) combining basic perceptual linear prediction

(PLP), RASTA-PLP, and modulation spectrograms. They also used a weighted finite state transducer (WFST) as in Mohri et al. (2002), and compared large-vocabulary connected speech recognition (LVCSR) with keyword-spotting (KWS) approaches to cope with hesitation, repetition or other vocal irregularities and to test whether the subjects were able to think of the right word (to assess for aphasia). They found KWS was the best approach, using the average of the top six posterior probabilities at each point in time as the "background" score as in Pinto et al. (2007). Overall performance was "promising" but there were considerable differences in performance between speakers.

The PEAKS system described in Maier et al. (2009) has already been implemented as an on-line tool. In their paper, they claim that their method "allows quantifying the intelligibility also in severely disturbed voices and speech." although this conclusion seems to be based on a database which only included a very small number of severely unintelligible speakers.

References

Accardo A, Fabbro F, Mumolo E (1992) Analysis of normal and pathological voices via short-time fractal dimension. In: Proceedings of annual international conference of the IEEE engineering in medicine and biology society, vol 14, pp 1270–1271

Alpan A, Schoentgen J, Maryn Y, Grenez F, Murphy P (2009) Cepstral analysis of vocal dysperiodicities in disordered connected speech. In: Proceedings of INTERSPEECH-2009, pp 959–962

Askenfelt A, Hammarberg B (1986) Speech waveform perturbation analysis: a perceptual-acoustical comparison of seven measures. J Speech Hearing Res 29:50–64

Awan SN, Scarpino SE (2004) Measures of vocal F0 from continuous speech samples: an inter-program comparison. J Speech Lang Pathol Audiol 28:122–131

Baken RI (1987) Clinical measurement of speech and voice. College Hill Press, Boston

Carmichael J, Wan V, Green P (2008) Combining neural network and rule-based systems for dysarthria diagnosis. In: Proceedings of INTERSPEECH-2008, pp 2226–2229

Castillo-Guerra E, Lovey DF (2003) A modern approach to dysarthria classification. In: 25th Annual Conference of the IEEE Engineering in Medicine and Biology Society, vol 3, 2257–2260. doi:10.1109/IEMBS.2003.1280248

Dahl GE, Yu D, Deng L, Acero A (2012) Context-dependent pre-trained deep neural networks for large vocabulary speech recognition. IEEE Trans Audio, Speech Lang Process 20(1):30–42. doi:10.1109/TASL.2011.2134090

de Krom G (1994) Consistency and reliability of voice quality ratings for different types of speech fragments. J Speech Hearing Res 37(5):965–1000

de Krom G (1995) Some spectral correlates of pathological breathy and rough voice quality for different types of vowel fragments. J Speech Hearing Res 38:794–811

Dibazar AA, Narayanan S, Berger TW (2002) Feature analysis for automatic detection of pathological speech. Eng Med and Biol 2002. In: Proceedings of the 24th annual conference and annual fall meeting of the biomedical engineering society EMBS/BMES, vol 1, pp 182–183. doi:10.1109/IEMBS.2002.1134447

Droppo J, Acero A (2010). In: IEEE international conference on acoustics speech and signal processing ICASSP-2010, pp 4358–4361. doi:10.1109/ICASSP.2010.5495652

Ganapathiraju A, Hamaker JE, Picone J (2004) Applications of support vector machines to speech recognition. IEEE Trans Signal Process 52(8):2348–2355. doi:10.1109/TSP.2004. 831018

Gunn SR (1998) Support vector machines for classification and regression. School of Electronics and Computer Science technical report, University of Southampton

Haderlein T, Zorn D, Steidl S, Nöth E, Shozakai M, Schuster M (2006) Visualization of voice disorders using the Sammon transform. In: Proceedings of the 9th international conference on text, speech and dialogue (TSD '06). Lecture notes in computer science, vol 4188, pp 589–596

Hariharan M, Paulraj MP, Yaacob S (2010) Time-domain features and probabilistic neural network for the detection of vocal fold pathology. Malays J Comput Sci 23(1):60–67

Henríquez P, Alonso JB, Ferrer MA, Travieso CM, Godino-Llorente JI, Díaz-de-María F (2009) Characterization of healthy and pathological voice through measures based on nonlinear dynamics. IEEE Trans Audio Speech Lang Process 17(6):1186–1195

Horii Y (1979) Fundamental frequency perturbation observed in sustained phonation. J Speech Hearing Res 22:5–19

Hosom JP, Shriberg L, Green JR (2004) Diagnostic assessment of childhood apraxia of speech using automatic speech recognition (ASR) methods. J Med Speech Lang Pathol 12(4):167–171

Kumar A, Mullick SK (1990) Attractor dimension, entropy and modelling of speech time series. Electron Lett 26(21):1790–1791

Llerena C, Alvarez L, Ayllon D (2011) Pitch detection in pathological voices driven by three tailored classical pitch detection algorithms. In: Recent advances in signal processing, computational geometry and systems theory. Proceeding of the ISCGAV'11 and ISTASC'11, pp 113–118

Maier A, Haderlein T, Eysholdt U, Rosanowski F, Batliner A, Schuster M, Nöth E (2009) PEAKS—a system for the automatic evaluation of voice and speech disorders. Speech Commun 51(5):425–437. doi:10.1016/j.specom.2009.01.004

Maier A, Haderlein T, Stelzle F, Nöth E, Nkenke E, Rosanowski F, Schützenberger A, Schuster M (2010) Automatic speech recognition systems for the evaluation of voice and speech disorders in head and neck cancer. EURASIP J Audio Speech Music Process. doi:10.1155/2010/926951

Malyska N, Quatieri TF, Sturim D (2005) Automatic dysphonia recognition using biologically inspired amplitude-modulation features. In: IEEE international conference on acoustics, speech, and. signal processing ICASSP-2005, pp 873–876

Markaki M, Stylianou Y (2009) Using modulation spectra for voice pathology detection and classification. In: Proceedings of the IEEE conference on engineering in medicine and biology society 2009, pp 2514–2517

Markaki M, Stylianou Y, Arias-Londono JD, Godino-Llorente JI (2010) Dysphonia detection based on modulation spectral features and cepstral coefficients. In Proceedings of ICASSP-2010, pp 5162–5165. doi:10.1109/ICASSP.2010.5495020

Middag C, Martens J-P, van Nuffelen G, de Bodt M (2009) Automated intelligibility assessment of pathological speech using phonological features. EURASIP J Adv Signal Process. doi:10.1155/2009/629030

Moakes PA, Beet S (1994) Analysis of non-linear speech generating dynamics. In Proceedings of 3rd international conference on spoken language processing (ICSLP 94), pp 1039–1042

Mohri M, Pereira F, Riley M (2002) Weighted finite-state transducers in speech recognition. Comput Speech Lang 16:69–88

Muhammad G, Mesallam TA, Malki KH, Farahat M, Alsulaiman M (2011) Formant analysis in dysphonic patients and automatic Arabic digit speech recognition. BioMed Eng OnLine 10:41. doi:10.1186/1475-925X-10-41

Padrell-Sendra J, Martin-Iglesias D, Diaz-de-Maria F (2006) Support vector machines for continuous speech recognition. In: Proceedings of the 14th European signal processing conference EUSIPCO-2006. http://www.eurasip.org/Proceedings/Eusipco/Eusipco2006/papers/1568981563.pdf. Accessed 16 Feb 2012

Parsa V, Jamieson DG (2001) Acoustic discrimination of pathological voice: sustained vowels versus continuous speech. J Speech Lang Hear Res 44:327–339

Pinto J, Lovitt A, Hermansky H (2007) Exploiting phoneme similarities in hybrid HMM-ANN keyword spotting. In Proceedings of INTERSPEECH-2007, pp 1817–1820

Pompili A, Abad A, Trancoso I, Fonseca J, Martins IP, Leal G, Farrajota L (2011) An on-line system for remote treatment of aphasia. In: Proceedings of 2nd workshop on speech and language processing for assistive technologies (SLPAT). http://www.inesc-id.pt/pt/indicadores/Ficheiros/7415.pdf. Accessed 16 Feb 2012

Reilly RB, Moran R, Lacy PD (2004) Voice pathology assessment based on a dialogue system and speech analysis. In Proc Amer Assoc Artif Intell Fall Symp Dialogue Syst Health Commun 104–109

Ringeval F, Demouy J, Szaszák G, Chetouani M, Robel L, Xavier J, Cohen D, Plaza M (2010) Automatic intonation recognition for the prosodic assessment of language-impaired children. IEEE Trans Audio, Speech, and Lang Process 19(5):1328–1342. doi:10.1109/TASL.2010.2090147

Salhi L, Mourad T, Cherif A (2010) Voice disorders identification using multilayer neural network. Int Arab J Inf Technol 7(2):177–185

Sammon JW (1969) A nonlinear mapping for data structure analysis. IEEE Trans Comput 18:401–409

Silva DG, Oliveira LC, Andrea M (2009) Jitter estimation algorithms for detection of pathological voices. EURASIP J Adv Signal Process 1–10. doi:10.1155/2009/567875

Steidl S, Stemmer G, Hacker C, Nöth E (2004) Adaption in the pronunciation space for non-native speech recognition. In Proc Int Conf on Spoken Lang Process ICSLP 318–321

Tsanas A, Little MA, McSharry PE, Spielman J, Ramig LO (2012) Novel speech signal processing algorithms for high-accuracy classification of Parkinson's disease. IEEE Trans Biomed Eng 59(5):1264–1271

Chapter 6
Novel Approaches

Abstract There are many avenues of research in this area which have still not been explored in any depth. Many of the techniques investigated during the history of speech and speaker recognition have fallen into obscurity because of their sensitivity to the very features of the speech signal which are likely to be the most helpful in diagnosis of speech disorders. One method, Multi-step Adaptive Flux Interpolation (MAFI), was developed by the authors of this book, and this chapter describes a pilot study which has applied features which were discarded in the original speech recognition and coding applications, to the identification of dysarthria and apraxia of speech (AOS). We compare this with an investigation of statistics derived from phonetic forced-alignment using hidden Markov models.

Keywords Adaptive flux interpolation · Dynamics of disordered speech · Hellinger distance · Score histograms

As examples of previously untried techniques for analysing disordered speech, this chapter presents a preliminary study we conducted using a minimal dataset, applying two novel methods intended to discriminate between normal and dysarthric speech, and apraxia of speech.

One method used statistics obtained from an HMM-based alignment, while the other used a technique originally developed for speech recognition and coding (Multi-step Adaptive Flux Interpolation, or MAFI). By adapting MAFI to reflect features related to the dynamics of the speech signal, we hoped to be able to discriminate between speakers with dysarthria and dyspraxia.

The aim of this study was to investigate the feasibility of methods based on extended samples of natural speech, collected under varying recording conditions, without tight control of recording procedures, and without the need for expert intervention in the preparation or manipulation of the recorded utterances.

6.1 The Data

This study was based on a very small dataset, since it was designed merely as a preliminary feasibility study, and to guide us in the choice of data for a subsequent full-scale investigation. We used data collected from three dysarthric speakers (one male and two female), one female dyspraxic speaker, and two other normal female speakers: one speaking the same text as the dysarthric speakers, "The Grandfather Passage" (Darley et al. 1975), and one who prompted the dyspraxic speaker with words and short phrases to be spoken. Thus we had normal and disordered versions of two distinct sets of utterances, but the words spoken by the dysarthric speakers were not the same as those spoken by the apraxic speaker.

For the dyspraxic speech, we used an existing speech recording from a cassette tape made in a quiet environment, but with significant levels of 'mains hum'. In order to remove any bias in the results due to this hum, all the data, including the HMM training data, was filtered to remove all frequencies below 300 Hz.

6.2 Phonetic Score Histograms

The first of the systems described here was inspired primarily by Green and Carmichael (2004), which investigated a feature which they termed the "goodness of fit" (GOF) of the speech to the HMM. Initially they evaluated this feature over a complete utterance, but went on to observe that GOF figures calculated separately for syllable-initial consonants appeared to be a more sensitive indicator of dysarthria. Their stated aim was to develop "an automated isolated-word intelligibility metric system designed to improve the scoring consistency and reliability of the Frenchay Dysarthria Assessment Test".

However, for the purposes of this study, our interest lies not in emulating human perception of intelligibility, but in mathematically discriminating between dysarthria, dyspraxia, and normal speech. We also require that any solution we devise, must not require expert recording or analysis skills. Thus we considered statistics of phoneme-level segments, but did not rely on identification of the phonemes in question or the positions of those segments within words, syllables or sentences.

We used Hidden Markov Models (HMMs) to align phonetic transcriptions with recorded utterances, to investigate the variation of 'log phoneme likelihood' without any manual phonetic segmentation or labelling of the speech. This parameter is produced as a by-product of alignment or recognition, and is known to increase in proportion to the duration of the phonemes, so the values were normalised by dividing by the respective durations.

In this study, the words spoken were all known a priori, so there was no need to perform recognition per se. Instead, we obtained the log phoneme probabilities by forced alignment of the speech with the phoneme sequences predicted by a simple

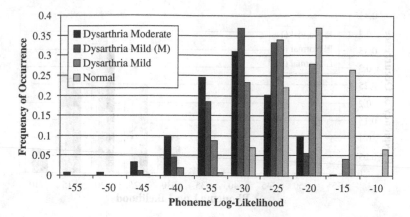

Fig. 6.1 Normalised histograms of 'normalised phoneme log-likelihoods' for different degrees of dysarthria: normal, mild, and moderate. All speakers were female apart from the one denoted (M). All values are based on analysis of the 'Grandfather Passage'. The peak of each distribution is further to the *left*, the more severe the impairment

dictionary-lookup. In any ultimate solution, the same parameters could be extracted from the results of large-vocabulary continuous speech recognition (LVCSR) system, or from word-level transcriptions and dictionary look-up.

Our system used a linear prediction (LP) cepstrum front-end, context-independent phoneme (monophone) HMMs with four 'left-to-right' states per phoneme and one-state skips, and with four Gaussian mixtures per state. The HMMs were trained using a large ad-hoc database of Southern British English speakers.

Having calculated a 'normalised phoneme log-likelihood' score for each phoneme uttered, we formed histograms of these scores separately for each speaker: normal, dysarthric, or dyspraxic. Because the dyspraxic recordings had been made with different protocols and equipment, we will discuss them separately, later.

6.2.1 Dysarthria Results

Visual examination of the dysarthria histograms (Fig. 6.1) shows a clear relationship between the degree of dysarthria and the normalised phoneme log-likelihood. The more severe the dysarthria, the more negative (further left) the peak of the respective histogram.

To confirm that these observations are not merely due to random variation from one utterance to another, Fig. 6.2 shows the same information but separately for three distinct readings of the 'Grandfather Passage' by a normal female speaker:

Thus, the peak of the HMM score histogram does indeed appear to indicate the degree of dysarthria. The shape of the distributions' low-end tails also provides a

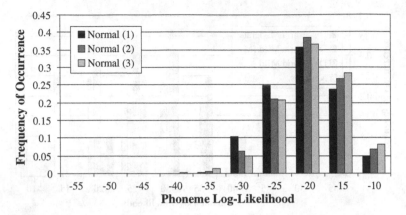

Fig. 6.2 Normalised histograms of 'normalised phoneme log-likelihoods' for three normal female utterances of the 'Grandfather Passage'. The peaks of all these distributions fall within the same histogram bin

potential cue to impairment severity: that of the moderate dysarthria distribution is higher and extends further than the normal speech, indicating that a significant number of phonemes may be pronounced very abnormally.

6.2.2 Dyspraxia Results

A similar analysis of the apraxia of speech results was performed separately because the relevant speech recordings were phonetically distinct from the dysarthric speech, above. The histograms are show in Fig. 6.3. Despite the recording conditions, the speakers, and both the phonetic and lexical content of the utterances being completely different, the 'normal' histogram from Fig. 6.3 is indistinguishable from those in Fig. 6.2. This suggests that these statistics of normalised phoneme log-probability should indeed be robust in real-world applications, being largely unaffected by differences in speaker identity, lexical and phonetic content, and recording procedures.

The observed differences between normal and dyspraxic speech were very small. There were slightly more very poor matches with dyspraxic speech (the lower tail of the dyspraxic histogram was noticeably raised), but based on such small dataset it is not possible to say if that difference is statistically significant.

6.2.3 Quantitative Comparison of HMM Score Histograms

To investigate exactly what can be reliably identified from these HMM score histograms, we need to be able to compare one with another and quantify the

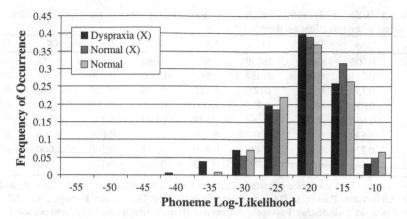

Fig. 6.3 Normalised histograms of 'normalised phoneme log-likelihoods' for one normal and one dyspraxic set of female utterances of diagnostic short phrases and words, marked with an (X), and one corresponding histogram for a different normal female speaker reading the 'Grandfather Passage'. The differences in the means and standard deviations of these distributions are statistically insignificant, but the lower tail of the dyspraxic histogram is clearly raised, relative to both the normal histograms

differences between them. Some such methods provide a measure which is both symmetrical (Eq. 6.1) and obeys the triangle inequality (Eq. 6.2):

$$D(a, b) = D(b, a) \tag{6.1}$$

$$D(a, b) \leq D(a, c) + D(b, c) \tag{6.2}$$

The triangle inequality is relevant here, because we intend to compare one histogram with two or more reference histograms, representing each of the reference conditions and/or severities. It is therefore intuitively helpful if the distance between two reference points, $D(a,b)$, is less than or equal to the sum of the distances between the unknown point, c, and the two references: $D(a,c) + D(b,c)$.

One measure which satisfies these conditions is the Hellinger distance, which can be expressed:

$$D_H(H_a, H_b) = \sqrt{1 - \sum \sqrt{H_a(i).H_b(i)}} \tag{6.3}$$

where $H_a(i)$ and $H_b(i)$ are the normalised values from bin i of histogram a and histogram b, respectively. The normalisation ensures that the elements of the histograms have the form of probability densities, such that Eqs. 6.4 and 6.5 are satisfied:

$$0 \leq H_x(i) \leq 1; \ \forall i; \ x = a, b \tag{6.4}$$

$$\sum_i H_x(i) = 1 \tag{6.5}$$

Table 6.1 Hellinger distances between the normalised phoneme log-probability distances mentioned in the preceding sections

	DA+	DM−	DA−	N1	N2	N3	NX	DX
DA+	0.000	0.243	0.339	0.658	0.686	0.679	0.729	0.611
DM-	0.243	0.000	0.354	0.664	0.706	0.708	0.747	0.655
DA−	0.339	0.354	0.000	0.415	0.460	0.467	0.498	0.392
N1	0.658	0.664	0.415	0.000	0.128	0.196	0.130	0.233
N2	0.686	0.706	0.460	0.128	0.000	0.148	0.113	0.220
N3	0.679	0.708	0.467	0.196	0.148	0.000	0.160	0.176
NX	0.729	0.747	0.498	0.130	0.113	0.160	0.000	0.228
DX	0.611	0.655	0.392	0.233	0.220	0.176	0.228	0.000

Abbreviations: *DA+* moderate dysarthria (female, Grandfather Passage), *DM−* mild dysarthria (male, Grandfather Passage), *DA−* mild dysarthria (female, Grandfather Passage), *N1*, *N2*, *N3* normal (female, Grandfather Passage), *NX* normal (female, diagnostic words and phrases), *DX* dyspraxic (female, diagnostic words and phrases)

Thus the Hellinger distance compares two discrete probability densities, and also has the convenient property that it lies between zero and one, with zero denoting that both normalised histograms are identical, and 'one' indicating that they are statistically unrelated.

6.2.4 Log-Probability Histogram Distances

Table 6.1 shows the Hellinger distances between the various histograms described above. The table is, of course, symmetrical because of the inherent symmetry of Hellinger distances. Abbreviations have been used instead of the condition, in order to keep the table compact.

As would be expected, the distances between all the normal speech histograms (N1, N2, N3, and NX), regardless of the words spoken, are small (<0.20). However, normal-to-dysarthric (DA+, DM−, DA−) distances are larger (>0.41), and increase with severity (>0.67 for moderate dysarthria, DA+).

Like most other standard measures, Hellinger distances are insensitive to small bumps in the tails of any distributions, and are primarily affected by differences in shape and position of the peaks. Thus the normal-to-dyspraxia (DX) distances are slightly greater than normal-to-normal distances, but still small (<0.24). The dyspraxic histogram is closer to the normal histograms than even the mild dysarthric ones.

Fig. 6.4 Lines of acoustic flow superimposed on a broad-band spectrogram of the word 'greasy'. The *white* lines show the movement of the features in the spectrogram between one frame and the next

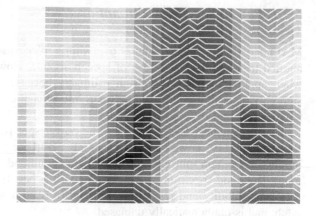

6.3 Multi-Step Adaptive Flux Interpolation

Moore et al. (1984) proposed the concept of "acoustic flow" in speech. This is a simple calculation based on power spectra taken from successive segments of a speech signal. It warps one power spectrum estimate to match the next using dynamic programming to optimise the warping, and so allows frequency-domain features to be tracked as they evolve over time (Fig. 6.4).

In Baghai-Ravary and Beet (1998) we extended this idea to identify segments of the speech signal which could be reconstructed, using lines of acoustic flow derived solely from the spectra at either end of the segment. We termed the resulting algorithm "Multi-step Adaptive Flux Interpolation", and successfully applied it to speech recognition, as well as speech and image coding.

MAFI allows us to quantify the number and abruptness of acoustic changes in a spoken passage. It is superior to piecewise-stationary models such as conventional variable frame-rate (VFR) coding scheme, in that it can identify a phonetic 'glide' as a single segment, without needing any special knowledge of what that segment may represent phonetically. The MAFI segments are generally of comparable size to, but not exactly the same as, traditional phonetic segments.

Thus MAFI provides statistics loosely related to the information extracted in papers such as Lindblom et al. (2009) regarding formant movements, but in an overall summary yet quantitative fashion, without explicit extraction of formants or any other discrete features.

MAFI provides two robust measures of the speech dynamics: one is the amount of movement in the frequency domain within each segment, while the other is the duration of the segment. The dynamics parameter is roughly proportional to the segment duration, so it is best normalised accordingly.

6.3.1 *Power Spectrum Estimation*

MAFI can yield some advantages over simple piecewise-stationary models when applied to most representations of speech signals. However, it is most effective when applied to power spectrum estimates because the formants often move smoothly, and almost linearly, between one phonetic 'target frequency' and the next.

There are many ways to estimate the power spectrum of a signal. In Baghai-Ravary et al. (1994) we compared a number of these methods, including periodograms, maximum entropy, and maximum likelihood, spectrograms. The maximum likelihood spectrum was found to give the best trade-off between clarity of formants, stability and resolution. It could also be made immune to changes in pitch, and is mathematically unbiased.

Thus, for the purposes of the current study, we used Maximum Likelihood power spectra evaluated on an ERB frequency scale (Moore and Glasberg 1987), with 24 ms time windows, one frame every 8 ms (a 3:1 overlap between successive frames), and 12th order linear prediction analysis (allowing for up to six peaks in the spectrum within the 8 kHz Nyquist band).

6.3.2 *MAFI Dynamics Parameters*

The MAFI analysis of dyspraxic speech is summarised in Fig. 6.5. This also shows a linear regression line, relating AFI dynamics and segment duration. The parameters of that line ('Offset' and 'Slope'), together with the Pearson correlation coefficient, R^2, provide a compact summary of the data's dynamic characteristics. The R^2 value is 'one' if there is a perfect straight-line fit, or 'zero' if there is no correlation.

This analysis was repeated for all the other recordings. The resulting linear regression parameters are illustrated in Figs. 6.6 and 6.7, showing differences between the data sets, and indicating any ability to discriminate between conditions and measure their severity.

In Fig. 6.6, the two 'diagnostic short phrases and words' (X) data sets are clustered together, some distance above all the other points. This suggests that the 'Slope' parameter is responding more to the text being spoken or some detail of the recording procedure, than any speech impairment or indeed, speaker identity.

Thus it appears that disordered speech exhibits slightly higher 'Slope' than normal speech, while 'Offset' clearly differentiates dysarthric speech, and to a lesser extent, dyspraxic, from normal speech.

The remaining parameter, the Pearson correlation coefficient is shown in Fig. 6.7 again with the 'Offset' as the horizontal axis. In this plot, the normal Grandfather Passage data sets are again clustered together in the bottom right-hand corner, but the normal 'diagnostic short phrases and words' point indicates a

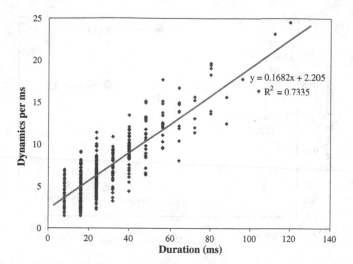

Fig. 6.5 Scatter plot showing MAFI dynamics parameter vs. segment duration for dyspraxic utterance of 'diagnostic short phrases and words', with the linear regression line with slope of 0.1682 and offset of 2.205. The Pearson correlation coefficient, R^2, is 0.7335, suggesting that the slope and offset of the linear regression line do indeed characterise a large part of the variation in the 'dynamics per ms' figure

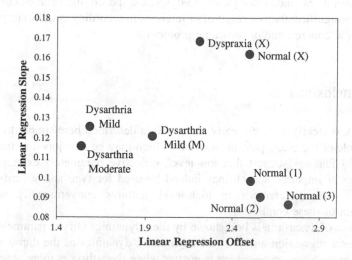

Fig. 6.6 Two linear regression parameters (slope and offset) derived from MAFI dynamics and segment durations. The utterances marked (X) were of 'diagnostic short phrases and words', while the others were of the 'Grandfather Passage'. All speakers were female apart from the one marked (M), and Normal (1) (2) and (3) were different instances recorded by the same speaker, with slightly different recording procedures

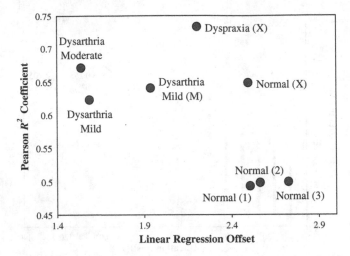

Fig. 6.7 Linear regression parameters (Pearson correlation coefficient and offset) derived from MAFI dynamics and segment durations

Pearson correlation significantly lower than the dyspraxic speech, being virtually the same as the dysarthric data. Thus the Pearson correlation appears to be the only of these parameters which is more sensitive to dyspraxia than dysarthria.

Although it responds more clearly to dyspraxic speech, the Pearson correlation also varies significantly as a result of differences in recording conditions, phonetic or linguistic content, and/or recording protocol.

6.4 Conclusions

This work is clearly at a very early stage, and is described here simply to provide an example of the many possible methods which may be developed in the future. Our initial findings suggest that low-level, objective parameters extracted from recordings of impaired speech may indeed be used for type and severity differentiation, without reference to high-level features conventionally used for assessment of these conditions.

Presence of dysarthria is best shown by the 'Dynamics Offset' parameter of the MAFI linear regression analysis (the asymptotic dynamics as the duration of the segment approaches zero—which is greater when dysarthria is more severe).

Severity of dysarthria is well indicated by both the 'Hellinger Distances' of log HMM probability data and the 'Pearson Correlation' of the AFI data.

The lower tails and the peaks of the HMM log probability distributions of impaired speech extend to more negative values than for normal speech. The Hellinger distances between normal and severely impaired speech are larger than those between speech of the same severity.

The Pearson correlation is higher for impaired speech, indicating that the speech is less controlled and influenced more by deterministic properties of the speech production process than by conscious control of the articulators by the speaker.

The analysis of dyspraxia is less clear-cut but possible differentiating cues are the combination of 'Dynamics Offset' and 'Pearson Correlation' of the AFI parameters, as may the be presence of a low HMM phoneme probability 'bump'.

As mentioned previously, the objective parameters explored in this paper, and their application, are at a very early stage of development. The next step should be to run our analyses on large datasets of dyspraxic and dysarthric speech and on different sub-types and severities, in order to refine the application and establish thresholds.

A further step would be to investigate the extent to which the discriminatory properties of MAFI correlate with clinical auditory assessment of intelligibility and impairment severity. An investigation of any differences between automatic and manual approaches could yield insights which might improve both automatic and manual assessment and diagnosis.

It is anticipated that any subsequent full-scale investigation would lead to significantly different conclusions, and the development of quite different methods, albeit with a similar underlying philosophy.

References

Baghai-Ravary L, Beet SW, Tokhi MO (1994) Removing redundancy from some common representations of speech. Proc Inst Acoust 16(5):467–474

Baghai-Ravary L, Beet SW (1998) Multistep coding of speech parameters for compression. IEEE Trans Speech Audio Process 6(5):435–444

Darley FL, Aronson AE, Brown JR (1975) Motor speech disorders. W. B Saunders, Philadelphia

Green P, Carmichael J (2004) Revisiting dysarthria assessment intelligibility metrics. In: Proceedings of INTERSPEECH-2004, pp 485–488

Lindblom B, Krull D, Hartelius L, Schalling E (2009) Formant transitions in normal and disordered speech: an acoustic measure of articulatory dynamics. In: Proceedings of FONETIK 2009, pp 18–23

Moore BCJ, Glasberg BR (1987) Formulae describing frequency selectivity as a function of frequency and level, and their use in calculating excitation patterns. Hearing Res 28:209–225

Moore RK, Tomlinson MJ, Beet SW (1984) The acoustic flow of speech. Proc Inst Acoust 6(4):241–248

Chapter 7
The Future

Abstract Some comments regarding future directions and developments in the field. In this section we attempt to summarise the most important issues surrounding current research in the area of identification and characterisation of disordered speech, and to indicate some promising avenues for future research.

Keywords Discrimination between disorders · Improved robustness · Mildly-disordered speech · Realistic evaluation · Unconstrained speech

Numerous automatic aids for diagnosis and monitoring of speech disorders have been proposed since the early 1990s. They have been based on a wide range of speech processing techniques, reflecting the general development of speech technology over that period.

However, the scope of research in this area has been strongly influenced by the availability of, and ease of recording new, samples of the different forms of speech disorder, as well as the relative difficulties of the tasks to be performed by the respective systems. For example, detection of a generic speech disorder is much easier than the discrimination between, say, different forms of dysarthria, and so many more techniques have been proposed for dysarthria detection, than for differential diagnosis between the different forms of dysarthria: flaccid, spastic, ataxic, etc., or between dysarthria and other disorders.

It seems likely that this tendency will continue for some time, despite the fact that performance on generic speech disorder/dysarthria detection has already exceeded the level at which the most commonly-used evaluation data (an age-and-gender balanced subset of the MEEI database) can differentiate between the best reported methods.

L. Baghai-Ravary and S. W. Beet, *Automatic Speech Signal Analysis for Clinical*   65
Diagnosis and Assessment of Speech Disorders, SpringerBriefs in Speech Technology,
DOI: 10.1007/978-1-4614-4574-6_7, © The Author(s) 2013

7.1 Evaluation

To adequately differentiate between the best of the current methods, it is imperative that cross-validation should become the de-facto standard for evaluation. Although the MEEI database is probably the single largest contribution to standardisation in this field, it was recorded many years ago and is fast becoming inadequate for evaluation of state-of-the-art algorithms, where detection of dysarthria, for example, can produce so few errors that the confidence with which the methods can be compared is inadequate.

There are some obvious limitations in the MEEI data, which need to be addressed to allow further progress:

1. There is an in-built inconsistency between the MEEI "normal" and "disordered" speech, quite apart from the differences in the original utterances (sample rates, durations of sustained phonation, and fixed duration of the Rainbow Passage utterances, at the very least). This means there are additional cues available to an automatic algorithm based on this data, which would not be available in "real-world" applications.
2. There is a scarcity of mildly disordered speech in the MEEI database, again making the detection of speech disorders unrealistically easy.
3. Although the database does contain examples of a good number of different speech disorders, many of the finer distinctions between specific variants of each disorder are not adequately represented. Hence their detection, or discrimination between them, cannot be adequately assessed.

All these shortcomings introduce factors which may have contributed to the observation that assessments using this database tend to be around 10 % absolute better than those on independent data.

Thus there is a pressing need for a comprehensive standardised database, collected specifically for the purpose of evaluation of automatic diagnostic aids. Some recently-collected alternatives, such as the "Universal Access" database, are starting to fill this gap, but there is still no single database which is suitable for the evaluation of all the systems being proposed.

The ideal database would require a very large-scale data collection exercise, covering the gamut of all common speech disorders, with varying degrees of severity and with non-disordered speech as well, all recorded with a consistent protocol and with good quality-control to ensure that there were no systematic differences between the different classes of speech.

To be of use in evaluating aids for differential diagnosis, the database would need to be designed such that, for each pair of conditions, pre-defined subsets of the respective conditions' recordings were specified, and each pair of subsets would be matched for distributions of gender, dialect and age. Clearly these subsets would need to be different for different pairs of conditions, and in order to provide a matching distribution for all possible disorders, the non-disordered speech would need to form a much larger part of the whole database than any other specific condition.

Current databases will still provide a valuable resource for training, both of clinicians and automatic systems, but a new 'ideal' database is needed to provide well-defined, demographically-balanced, and sufficiently large datasets for evaluation on disorder-detection, disorder-discrimination, and degree-of-disorder-estimation tasks.

7.2 Promising Topics for Future Research

In recent years, several papers have reported accuracies of dysarthria detection in excess of 99 %, based on the sustained phonation recordings from the MEEI database. It might appear from these results that there is little room for improvement in this field, but as suggested above, it is unlikely that the accuracies achieved on speech "in the wild" would be nearly so impressive. The effects of less controlled recording conditions, the presence of subjects with less clear-cut levels of disorder, or even combinations of multiple disorders, and the use of lossy encodings for storage and/or transmission of the data, will all reduce the effectiveness of such techniques.

Thus there are two directions of research which would continue this already successful theme

1. Improving the robustness of dysarthria detection to uncontrolled variations in the data-collection process.
2. Improving the ability to detect mildly-disordered dysarthric speech, or dysarthria in conjunction with other forms of speech disorder.

Other areas of research into automatic analysis of speech disorders have not yet produced such high levels of accuracy as dysarthria detection. Some depend on a higher level analysis of the speech signal (discriminating between apraxia of speech, stuttering, and normal disfluency for example), and this could well be the reason why less work has been reported in this area. Others ought not require these higher cognitive levels of analysis, but do need to be sensitive to more subtle cues in the characteristics of the speech signal: discrimination between dysarthria and simple dysphonia, for example.

These subtle cues could include features such as rhythm and intonation, which are, to some extent, correlated with statistics regarding the ranges of, and correlations between, syllable amplitudes and durations, and dynamic aspects of pitch. Although precise syllable timings can still be somewhat elusive, especially in spontaneous speech, it is quite possible to extract other robust features which are, at least loosely, related to syllable durations or pitch contours.

Similarly, other potentially fruitful areas of research include discrimination between similar disorders as well as different forms of the various disorders. Such discrimination will require significant breakthroughs in some cases, since most current models of speech production and perception are based around "normal" speech and simple phonetic and lexically-based representations.

When speech disorders are to be included in the equation, these models are inadequate because they do not allow for systematically incomplete, inaccurate, or otherwise atypical deviations from the norm (for example in stuttering, where partial phoneme sequences may be repeated, or in dysarthria, where the phonetic identity of the sounds may be distorted in specific ways pertinent only to specific varieties of the condition.

7.3 The Techniques Most Likely to Succeed

It has been repeatedly demonstrated in virtually all aspects of speech technology, that the most successful methods are those which can be trained or optimised automatically, based on large databases, analysed with the minimum of human intervention. Although experts can provide extremely valuable insights into the most important features of speech and language, they are notoriously inexact in their interpretation of those features and are unable to fully optimise their calculation or usage in automatic systems.

Thus it is probable that the most successful techniques will involve technologies such as support vector machines, discriminant analysis (whether linear or non-linear), radial basis function networks, multi-layer perceptrons, deep belief networks, and (of course) the many variants of hidden Markov models.

In the case of HMMs, there have been many advances in recent years, both in the structure of the models (continuous, discrete, semi-continuous, semi-hidden, etc.), and in the training procedures (maximum mutual information, minimum phone error, vocal tract length normalisation, and many others).

A number of these recent developments have been applied to disordered speech, but others have relatively untapped potential in this area. In some cases, the details of the procedures might need significant modification when the discrimination is ultimately between disorders of speech rather than phoneme sequences.

To be effective at discriminating between disorders, or to assess severity of higher-level disorders, new methods will be needed to characterise features of the speech which have not been required previously. They should be able to identify unusual duration or intonation patterns, as well as deviations from phonological and lexical norms. This latter requirement needs more sophisticated models of spoken language than the simple, albeit statistically robust, N-gram approach, which currently dominates the world of large-vocabulary speech recognition. Similarly, current models of intonation are still incomplete, and both the quantification and comparison of intonation patterns, and the determination of exactly what constitutes 'normality' in the first place, are problems which need much further effort to resolve.

Thus there is great scope for further work, both by applying existing techniques from the speech recognition and processing fields, and by developing new techniques which can highlight relevant aspects of the speech signals.

7.4 Practical Approaches

In finding new solutions to the problems described in this book, it is crucial to keep in mind the realities of the range of environments where the system might be applied. At the very least, this should include variations due to microphone placement, reverberation, and background noise.

Methods should also minimise errors due to mistakes or omissions when following any experimental protocol. There are two approaches to achieving this aim—either by making the protocol so simple and rigidly defined that deviations from it become vanishingly rare, or by making the protocol so flexible that unrestricted recordings of natural speech can be used.

Both of these approaches have clear problems. For the 'strict protocol' approach, the recording procedure becomes limited to collection of short words or even individual sounds (such as the sustained /a/ phonations which are known to be valuable in diagnosing dysarthria, but are of little relevance to apraxia of speech). For the 'flexible protocol' approach, the difficulty is simply shifted from enforcing adherence to the protocol, onto the subsequent analysis procedure: the recordings need to be analysed in ways which are immune to differences in phonetic, semantic, and even emotional content, and environmental factors, including the presence of other voices and noises. This is not fully achievable with current technology, but would be highly advantageous if 'higher-level' neurological disorders are to be successfully diagnosed.

So it appears that the greatest benefit to future remote diagnosis and telemonitoring will be provided by methods based around recordings of (broadly) unrestricted speech. The current methods which are closest to achieving this are those which require subjects to read extended passages, or repeat verbal prompts spoken by the clinician. However, the symptoms of conditions such as stuttering are known to be dependent on the emotional state and level of stress of the subject. Thus the severity of any condition, as it affects their day-to-day communication, can only be meaningfully assessed by analysing natural, spontaneous communication; not read or verbally prompted text.

To that end, it is highly desirable that more effort should be put into developing techniques for characterising both signal dynamics (independent of phonetic, lexical, and linguistic content), and the linguistic and para-linguistic, aspects of informally collected natural speech. Of these two approaches, the analysis of signal dynamics is much more straightforward, but advances in linguistic analysis of disordered speech could ultimately yield greater rewards.

7.5 Conclusion

Automatic characterisation of disordered speech is potentially of very great value, and could make use of many existing forms of speech technology. Much of that technology is already firmly established, and in daily use by the majority of the population of technologically developed countries.

However, despite the maturity of much of the underlying technology, 'automatic analysis of disordered speech' remains a field which is not fully explored. Impressively high accuracies have been obtained in artificial laboratory conditions, but the methods are frustratingly difficult to translate into robust and reliable clinical tools, suitable for day-to-day use. While accuracies in excess of 99 % are commonly quoted in scientific literature, real-world accuracies (even when recordings are closely controlled) are rarely in excess of 85 %, and substantially lower for more demanding tasks.

Thus there is still a great deal of scope for progress in this area. Because of the nature of the problem, much can be adapted from other fields of speech technology, but to date, relatively few researchers have explicitly focussed on speaker recognition as a source domain. This seems somewhat odd, in that it is the established application which has most in common with the identification and characterisation of speech disorders. In particular, likelihood normalisation and model-based compensation methods seem likely to yield parameters which could be useful in identifying unusual speaker characteristics.